PAIN NO MORE

7 Proven Secrets To End Chronic Pain

Second Edition

Dr. Joseph Jacobs, DPT, ACN

Second Edition, March 2025

Published by ASTR Institute
614 E HWY 50 #169, Clermont, FL 34711

ASTR

ASTRinstitute.com

Disclaimer

This book, authored by Dr. Joseph Jacobs and published by the ASTR Institute, is intended for informational purposes only and presents medical research findings. It is not a substitute for professional medical advice, diagnosis, or treatment. Dr. Joseph Jacobs, the ASTR Institute, and its affiliates do not endorse or assume responsibility for any specific medical treatments or procedures discussed in this book. We strongly advise readers to consult with their healthcare providers regarding the applicability of any aspects of the content to their own health and well-being.

The statements contained herein have not been evaluated by the Food and Drug Administration. The products mentioned are not designed to diagnose, cure, treat, or prevent any disease. Individual results may vary, and we cannot guarantee that you will achieve the same outcomes as those detailed in our case studies, testimonials, and treatment videos. Success varies per individual, and one person's results do not guarantee similar outcomes for another.

If you have medical concerns, consult with your healthcare provider, physician, or another qualified medical professional. Dr. Joseph Jacobs, the ASTR Institute, and their associated organizations and individuals disclaim any liability for actions, services, or products acquired through this book, our videos, website, or any of our media channels.

Table of Contents

- Online Resources   V

- Triumph Over Trials: My Journey from Disability to Victory   1

- Case Studies   5

- 21 Medical Myths Debunked: What Your Doctor Got Wrong   15

- The Biopsychosocial Model: A Paradigm Shift in Health Care   38

- Navigating The Healing Journey: How Your Body Recovers Naturally 50

- 7 Proven Secrets

    1.   Posture and Body Mechanics   56

    2.   Inflammatory Foods   66

    3.   Stress Management   73

    4.   Fibrotic Tissue   80

    5.   Fascial Restriction   91

    6.   Behavior Modification   103

    7.   Vitamin, Mineral, and Hormonal Imbalances   107

- Conclusion   116

- Recommended Resources   120

- Glossary   125

- References   132

Online Resources

How to Access Online Resources

Throughout this book, you'll find barcodes that link to additional online resources. Here's how to use them:

1. Open the camera app on your smartphone.
2. Point the camera at the barcode.
3. A notification will appear with a link. Tap the notification to open the link in your browser.

Triumph Over Trials: My Journey from Disability to Victory

Triumph Over Trials

After my second cancer treatment, I was suffering from chronic fatigue, migraines, muscle and joint pain. I reached out to at least seven doctors, but I could not find relief. Unfortunately, they had two responses. First, they said my blood labs looked normal. I learned from my studies in nutrition that this happened because they did not order the correct labs to figure out the root cause of my issues. The second response was that I was a hopeless case. This made me realize that if I wanted to overcome my disability, I had to look for a solution on my own. It was a difficult time in my life. Due to my pain and fatigue, it used to take me 10 minutes just to walk from the living room to the bathroom, about 20 feet away. I was very depressed and angry because, at 30 years old, I was facing numerous health issues and had a poor quality of life without any answers.

I spent countless hours and years studying nutrition, psychology, behavioral modification, anatomy, physiology, ergonomics, and other medical topics in hopes of finding an answer. At the same time, I was frustrated that the techniques I learned in medical school only provided short-term results with no lasting relief. I tried what I learned in school, such as stretching, exercises, electrical stimulation, various massage techniques, manual therapy, joint mobilization, and myofascial release, but nothing provided long-term results. So,

I started to look at medical studies to guide me through this process. After reviewing over 16,000 medical research papers with assistance from medical students, I was shocked and disappointed by the results. Based on these studies, the following treatments either provided no pain reduction or only short-term pain reduction:
- NSAIDs
- Opioids
- Cortisone shots
- Exercises
- Stretching
- Massage
- Joint mobilization or manipulation
- Acupuncture

- Dry needling
- Instrument-assisted soft tissue mobilization

I have dedicated my life to researching all current traditional medical approaches to treating pain. I've found that the majority of these approaches primarily focus on relieving symptoms rather than addressing the root cause of the pain. The techniques I learned in school, still used in today's modern medical world, have their origins in ancient healing practices such as manipulation, massage, stretching, and exercise. These methods were used by the Romans, Greeks, and Egyptians to increase flexibility, strengthen muscles, and alleviate pain. Today's medicine has added treatments like cold, heat, electrical stimulation, and joint adjustment to this list. However, overwhelming evidence from published medical studies shows no promising long-term relief from any of these methods. For instance, one systematic review conducted by the University of Ottawa, Canada, which reviewed 270 research studies, concluded that the benefits of massage, acupuncture, and spine adjustment treatments were mostly evident immediately or shortly after treatment, then faded over time.

With compelling data like this, it is perplexing how we continue to treat patients with modalities that do not effectively address their long-term needs. Instead of focusing so much on the body's symptoms, we need to start questioning why these symptoms are present in the first place and why they keep returning. This question guided me through an intense investigative research process over five years. From this research, I concluded that there are seven aspects of chronic pain that, when treated simultaneously, can lead to long-term pain relief. I also found that the BioPsychosocial model is an effective treatment approach for long-term pain reduction. So, I studied the BioPsychosocial model in depth and realized that my medical education was lacking in nutrition knowledge. I spent thousands of hours reading and studying nutrition and bought any book that I felt could help me understand the body better.

During this time, my wife had chronic jaw pain due to stress at work. I tried everything I learned from school on her, but nothing provided long-term pain relief. One day she woke up with lockjaw, unable to speak or open her mouth.

Triumph Over Trials

She asked me to try anything. I told her that I had tried everything I knew, but nothing worked. So, I reached inside her mouth and experimented with several maneuvers. After a few minutes, she was able to open her mouth and was pain-free. I was dumbfounded and had no idea what had just happened. It took me several days to understand the physiology of the maneuvers I had performed. I then started experimenting with the same concept, applying it to the whole body to relieve both my pain and my patients' pain.

After several months of using my hands to implement the new maneuvers I had come up with, I realized I could not do that long-term. My hands were very sore, and I suffered from pain every night. I told my wife that this was not sustainable because I was in so much pain from using my hands. While patients were getting relief, I was suffering. My wife suggested that I use tools instead of my hands. So, I went to a hardware store and bought rubber, plastic, and metal to cut and design tools and devices to replace my hand maneuvers. Thankfully, this provided even faster results for my patients without me feeling soreness from working on them.

I was able to overcome my chronic fatigue and migraines by running comprehensive lab tests. These tests revealed several vitamin, mineral, and hormonal imbalances. Additionally, I overcame my chronic joint and muscle pain through the biopsychosocial (BPS) model and the tools and devices I invented. I also reinvented the biopsychosocial model to be implemented by a single healthcare provider and called it ASTR treatment. In the following chapters, I will share many tips that you can apply today to relieve your pain and begin your healing journey.

Case Studies

Case Studies

All case studies presented in this book demonstrate that the BPS model can be implemented by a single healthcare provider. Case studies and recorded live treatment videos are available online. Use the barcode or the following link to watch: https://advancedsofttissuerelease.com/treatment-videos-2/.

Case Study 10: 8 Years of Neck Pain

Diagnosis: Neck disc herniation from car accident
Symptoms: Sharp neck pain, right arm/shoulder dull aching pain, limited range of motion, and limited activities.
Previous Failed Treatments: Physical therapy and trigger point injection.
Length of Injury: 8 years.
Pain Level on a Scale of 0 to 10: 6-8/10.
Treatment: Treatment included releasing fibrotic tissue, addressing fascia restrictions, decreasing inflammation, improving ergonomics, implementing an anti-inflammatory diet, and addressing vitamin, mineral, and hormonal imbalances.
Outcome: Symptoms resolved.

Case Study 11: 1 Month of Neck Pain

Diagnosis: Neck pain after workout.
Symptoms: Constant dull/sharp neck and upper back pain
Previous Failed Treatments: Foam roller.
Length of Injury: 1 month.
Pain Level on a Scale of 0 to 10: 3-9/10.
Treatment: Treatment included releasing fibrotic tissue, addressing fascia restrictions, decreasing inflammation, improving ergonomics, and implementing

an anti-inflammatory diet.
Outcome: Symptoms resolved.

Case Study 12: 16 Years of Neck Pain

Diagnosis: Neck pain after car accident.
Symptoms: Neck and traps pain.
Previous Failed Treatments: Chiropractor, massage therapy, and physical therapy.
Length of Injury: 16 years.
Pain Level on a Scale of 0 to 10: 6-7/10.
Treatment: Treatment included releasing fibrotic tissue, addressing fascia restrictions, decreasing inflammation, improving ergonomics, and implementing an anti-inflammatory diet.
Outcome: Symptoms resolved.

Case Study 13: 10 Years of Neck and Shoulder Pain

Diagnosis: Neck and shoulder pain after car accident.
Symptoms: Neck pain, trapezius pain, muscle spasm, difficulty driving, difficulty sleeping, and limited shoulder flexion.
Previous Failed Treatments: 6 different physical therapists, 2 different chiropractors, and acupuncture.
Length of Injury: 10 years.
Pain Level on a Scale of 0 to 10: 3-10/10.
Treatment: Treatment included releasing fibrotic tissue, addressing fascia restrictions, decreasing inflammation, improving ergonomics, and implementing an anti-inflammatory diet.
Outcome: Symptoms resolved.

Case Study 14: 30 Years of Back Pain and Bilateral Leg Numbness

Diagnosis: Back pain after lifting a wheelchair.
Symptoms: Constant back pain, aching and stabbing, with radiation to bilateral

lower extremities, tingling, and numbness, limping stiff gait, and unable to sleep on bed.
Previous Failed Treatments: Back fusion surgery and physical therapy.
Length of Injury: 30 years.
Pain Level on a Scale of 0 to 10: 3-10/10.
Treatment: Treatment included releasing fibrotic tissue, addressing fascia restrictions, decreasing inflammation, improving ergonomics, implementing an anti-inflammatory diet, and addressing vitamin, mineral, and hormonal imbalances.
Outcome: Symptoms resolved.

Case Study 15: 7 Years of Back Pain and Leg Pain

Diagnosis: Back pain after car accidents.
Symptoms: Constant back pain, thigh/ leg pain, unable to sit up on bed, and very stiff back.
Previous Failed Treatments: back ablation surgery, a lot physical therapy, and a lot of massage therapy.
Length of Injury: 7 years.
Pain Level on a Scale of 0 to 10: 3-10/10.
Treatment: Treatment included releasing fibrotic tissue, addressing fascia restrictions, decreasing inflammation, improving ergonomics, implementing an anti-inflammatory diet.
Outcome: Symptoms resolved.

Case Study 16: 2 Years of Low Back Pain

Diagnosis: Low back pain.
Symptoms: Low back pain, muscle spasm, and numbness/ needle pain.
Previous Failed Treatments:
Length of Injury: 2 years.
Pain Level on a Scale of 0 to 10: 7-9/10.
Treatment: Treatment included releasing fibrotic tissue, addressing fascia

restrictions, decreasing inflammation, improving ergonomics, implementing an anti-inflammatory diet.
Outcome: Symptoms resolved.

Case Study 17: 10 Years of Migraines, Daily Headaches, and Jaw Pain

Diagnosis: Migraines and jaw pain.
Symptoms: Migraines; jaw, ear, temporal, face, and neck pain; constant daily headaches at 4/10 that increase throughout the day; teeth grinding.
Previous Failed Treatments: Dentist, neurologist, medication, migraine medications, massage therapy, chiropractor, acupuncture, and essential oils.
Length of Injury: 10 years.
Pain Level on a Scale of 0 to 10: 4-8/10.
Treatment: Treatment included releasing fibrotic tissue, addressing fascia restrictions, decreasing inflammation, improving ergonomics, and implementing an anti-inflammatory diet.
Outcome: Symptoms resolved.

Case Study 18: 4 Months of Migraines, Neck and Shoulder Pain

Diagnosis: Migraines & neck and shoulder Pain.
Symptoms: Migraines several times a week, neck and shoulder soreness, fatigue, sensitivity to light, nausea, migraine aura, and eye pressure.
Previous Failed Treatments: Medication and migraine medications.
Length of Injury: 4 months.
Pain Level on a Scale of 0 to 10: 4-5/10.
Treatment: Treatment included releasing fibrotic tissue, addressing fascia restrictions, decreasing inflammation, improving ergonomics, and implementing an anti-inflammatory diet.
Outcome: Symptoms resolved.

Case Study 19: 5 Years of Daily Tension Headaches, Neck, and Jaw Pain
Diagnosis: Daily tension headaches.
Symptoms: Daily headaches, blurry vision, jaw pain, neck pain, jaw clicks, and

throbbing head pain.
Previous Failed Treatments: Neurologist, ENT doctor, various physical therapists, chiropractor, neck specialist, botox shots, cortisone shots, muscle relaxers, and medication.
Length of Injury: 5 years.
Pain Level on a Scale of 0 to 10: 4-5/10.
Treatment: Treatment included releasing fibrotic tissue, addressing fascia restrictions, decreasing inflammation, improving ergonomics, and implementing an anti-inflammatory diet.
Outcome: Symptoms resolved.

Case Study 20: 2 Years of Tension Headaches
Diagnosis: Tension headaches.
Symptoms: Almost daily headaches and neck stiffness.
Previous Failed Treatments: medication.
Length of Injury: 2 years
Pain Level on a Scale of 0 to 10: 4-6/10.
Treatment: Treatment included releasing fibrotic tissue, addressing fascia restrictions, decreasing inflammation, improving ergonomics, and implementing an anti-inflammatory diet.
Outcome: Symptoms resolved.

Case Study 21: Locked Jaw and Migraines

Diagnosis: Locked jaw and migraines.
Symptoms: Locked jaw, migraines, face and neck pain, inability to chew, and inability to sleep.
Previous Failed Treatments: Dentist and medication.
Length of Injury: 1 week.
Pain Level on a Scale of 0 to 10: 9-10/10.
Treatment: Treatment included releasing fibrotic tissue, addressing fascia restrictions, decreasing inflammation, improving ergonomics, and implementing an anti-inflammatory diet.
Outcome: Symptoms resolved.

Case Studies

Case Study 22: 4 Years of Shoulder Stiffness and Pain

Diagnosis: Shoulder pain.
Symptoms: Shoulder pain increases with throwing and sports activities. Additional symptoms include shoulder stiffness and tightness, shoulder clicking, and shoulder instability.
Previous Failed Treatments: Physical therapy.
Length of Injury: 4 years.
Pain Level on a Scale of 0 to 10: 2/10.
Treatment: Treatment included releasing fibrotic tissue, addressing fascia restrictions, decreasing inflammation, improving ergonomics, and implementing an anti-inflammatory diet, and addressing vitamin, mineral, and hormonal imbalances.
Outcome: Symptoms resolved.

Case Study 23: 3 Years of Tennis Elbow

Diagnosis: Tennis elbow.
Symptoms: Almost daily headaches and neck stiffness.
Previous Failed Treatments: Ice, elbow braces and massage therapy.
Length of Injury: 3 years.
Pain Level on a Scale of 0 to 10: 3-7/10.
Treatment: Treatment included releasing fibrotic tissue, addressing fascia restrictions, decreasing inflammation, improving ergonomics, and implementing an anti-inflammatory diet and addressing vitamin, mineral, and hormonal imbalances.
Outcome: Symptoms resolved.

Case Study 24: 6 Months of Golfer's Elbow

Diagnosis: Golfer's elbow.
Symptoms: Left medial elbow pain that increases with lifting objects.
Previous Failed Treatments: Acupuncture, and massage therapy.
Length of Injury: 6 months.

Pain Level on a Scale of 0 to 10: 4/10.
Treatment: Treatment included releasing fibrotic tissue, addressing fascia restrictions, decreasing inflammation, improving ergonomics, and implementing an anti-inflammatory diet.
Outcome: Symptoms resolved.

Case Study 25: 2 Years of Trigger Finger

Diagnosis: Trigger finger.
Symptoms: Trigger finger with pain, locking, and stiffness; more locking in the morning.
Previous Failed Treatments: Physical therapy, massage, and diet change.
Length of Injury: 2 years.
Pain Level on a Scale of 0 to 10: 3-8/10.
Treatment: Treatment included releasing fibrotic tissue, addressing fascia restrictions, decreasing inflammation, improving ergonomics, and implementing an anti-inflammatory diet.
Outcome: Symptoms resolved.

Case Study 26: 1 Month of Carpal Tunnel Syndrome

Diagnosis: Carpal tunnel syndrome.
Symptoms: Sharp finger pain, numbness and tingling, and wrist pain. The pain increases with self-care activities and working.
Previous Failed Treatments: Medication, neurologist, and acupuncture.
Length of Injury: 1 month.
Pain Level on a Scale of 0 to 10: 7/10.
Treatment: Treatment included releasing fibrotic tissue, addressing fascia restrictions, decreasing inflammation, improving ergonomics, and implementing an anti-inflammatory diet.
Outcome: Symptoms resolved.

Case Study 27: 2 Years of Knee Stiffness and Pain

Case Studies

Diagnosis: Knee pain, medial and lateral meniscus tear.
Symptoms: Decreased knee range of motion, thigh muscle spasm, knee buckling, and knee instability.
Previous Failed Treatments: Physical therapy and pressure compression.
Length of Injury: 2 years.
Pain Level on a Scale of 0 to 10: 7/10.
Treatment: Treatment included releasing fibrotic tissue, addressing fascia restrictions, decreasing inflammation, improving ergonomics, and implementing an anti-inflammatory diet.
Outcome: Symptoms resolved.

Case Study 28: 5 Years of Morton's Neuroma

Diagnosis: Bilateral feet Morton's neuroma.
Symptoms: Bilateral feet pain with constant 5/10 pain, which increases with weight bearing. Symptoms started after bunion removal surgery, and the patient has a very stiff, limping gait.
Previous Failed Treatments: 5 different podiatrists, physical therapy, chiropractor, massage therapy, cortisone shots, foot orthotics, and special shoes.
Length of Injury: 5 years.
Pain Level on a Scale of 0 to 10: 5-9/10.
Treatment: Treatment included releasing fibrotic tissue, addressing fascia restrictions, decreasing inflammation, improving ergonomics, implementing an anti-inflammatory diet, and addressing vitamin, mineral, and hormonal imbalances.
Outcome: Symptoms resolved.

Case Study 29: 8 Years of Chronic Fatigue
Diagnosis: Chronic fatigue.
Symptoms: Chronic fatigue, tired, lethargic, very low energy, and hair thinning.
Previous Failed Treatments: physical therapy, vitamins and supplements.
Length of Injury: 8 Years.
Pain Level on a Scale of 0 to 10:
Treatment: Treatment included releasing fibrotic tissue, addressing fascia

Case Studies

restrictions, decreasing inflammation, improving ergonomics, implementing an anti-inflammatory diet, and addressing vitamin, mineral, and hormonal imbalances.

Outcome: Symptoms resolved.

For more case studies and live recorded treatments, use the barcode or the following link to watch: https://advancedsofttissuerelease.com/treatment-videos-2/.

21 Medical Myths Debunked: What Your Doctor Got Wrong

Chronic pain can be managed through various treatments that typically fall into one of two categories: 1. biomedical model (Western medicine) approaches, and 2. biopsychosocial approaches (either provided in a multidisciplinary approach or by a single healthcare provider). Biomedical model treatment approaches are utilized by medical doctors, osteopathic doctors, naturopathic doctors, chiropractors, physical therapists, occupational therapists, and acupuncturists. These approaches include opioids, NSAIDs, massage, manual therapy, acupuncture, steroid injections, spinal manipulation, stretching and exercises, dry needling, trigger point injections, and the use of Kinesio Tape along with other specialized tools.

This chapter will present research studies investigating the effectiveness of the biomedical model approach. We will examine the studies that investigated the efficacy of the biomedical model.

Is it better to use the biomedical model or the biopsychosocial (BPS) model to address chronic pain?

Before answering this question, we need to understand the different types of research studies available and determine which ones are the most reliable sources of information. This understanding will help us make the best clinical decisions based on thousands of studies.

The following overview of different types of research studies will help us select the right type of study. This, in turn, will enable us to make the best clinical decisions and choose the most effective treatment approach for chronic pain.

- **Randomized Controlled Trials (RCTs):** Participants are randomly assigned to either the treatment group or the control group. The treatment group receives the intervention being tested, while the control group receives a placebo or standard treatment. This randomization helps to eliminate bias, allowing researchers to determine the effectiveness and safety of a medical intervention.

- **Observational Studies:** Unlike RCTs, observational studies do not involve intervention by the researcher. Instead, they involve observing the effects of a risk factor, diagnostic test, treatment, or other intervention without trying to change who is or isn't exposed to it.
- **Cohort Studies:** These are observational studies that follow a group of people over time. Participants in these studies are chosen based on specific exposures (such as smoking) and then followed to see the outcomes they develop. Researchers can track if exposure is associated with a higher likelihood of certain health outcomes. Cohort studies can be prospective (following participants forward in time) or retrospective.
- **Case Reports:** Detailed presentations of a single patient's medical history, symptoms, diagnosis, treatment, and follow-up. Case reports are valuable for sharing unusual medical conditions or the effects of new treatments.
- **Meta-Analyses:** This type of research synthesizes data from multiple studies on the same subject. Meta-analyses use statistical techniques to combine results of eligible scientific studies. This provides a high level of evidence on the efficacy or safety of a treatment or an association, often influencing clinical practice and guidelines.
- **Systematic Reviews:** These reviews are comprehensive surveys of a topic. In them, all the primary studies of the highest level of evidence have been systematically identified, appraised, and then summarized according to an explicit and reproducible methodology. They often include meta-analyses to statistically analyze the data.

Advantages of Meta-Analyses and Systematic Reviews

Meta-analyses and systematic reviews are the most efficient types of research studies. They review several medical studies, saving time and effort in evaluating each individual study to reach a proper conclusion. Meta-analyses and systematic reviews are powerful research tools in the scientific community, offering several key benefits:

1. **Comprehensive Overview:** They provide a complete overview of existing research on a specific topic. By integrating findings from multiple studies, they identify general trends and conclusions.
2. **Increased Statistical Power:** By pooling data from several studies, meta-analyses increase the statistical power of the analysis. This enhances the reliability of the conclusions.
3. **Resolution of Discrepancies:** These reviews can help resolve conflicting results from different studies. This allows researchers to determine which factors may have contributed to discrepancies in outcomes.
4. **Evidence-Based Practice:** They are fundamental in guiding evidence-based practice, helping policymakers, clinicians, and other stakeholders make informed decisions based on the weight of multiple studies rather than a single source.
5. **Identification of Research Gaps:** Systematic reviews can reveal gaps in the current research. They provide guidance for future studies and highlight areas where further investigation is needed.
6. **Reduction of Bias:** A well-conducted systematic review follows a rigorous and predefined methodology. This helps reduce bias in the selection and analysis of studies included in the review.
7. **Time and Cost Efficiency:** By synthesizing existing studies, these reviews save time and resources. This prevents the need to conduct new research that may replicate already available findings
8. **Policy and Decision Making:** The comprehensive data provided by meta-analyses can support stronger and more accurate decision-making in healthcare, environmental policy, education, and other fields.
9. **Global Insights:** They often include studies from multiple countries. This provides insights that are globally relevant and can be applied in various cultural or regional contexts.
10. **Educational Value:** For students and new researchers, systematic reviews and meta-analyses serve as valuable educational resources. They help in understanding the scope of research on a particular topic and in learning about methodologies.

Is it better to use the biomedical model or the biopsychosocial (BPS) model to address chronic pain?

There are an overwhelming number of studies indicating that the biomedical treatment model either provides short-term pain reduction or no pain reduction. In some cases, the placebo effect performed better than the biomedical model due to the severe adverse effects of the biomedical model treatments.

The following section presents detailed research study findings. If you do not like to read <u>dry scientific information,</u> you can skip to the end of this chapter to read the conclusion.

The following section was sourced from several systematic reviews, meta-analyses, and literature reviews. One of the studies, titled "Evaluating the Effectiveness of Treatment Options for Pain," was published in the Orthopedic Research Journal. The research for this study involved a comprehensive literature search conducted across major databases including Medline, ScienceDirect, PubMed, Embase, Google Scholar, Cinahl, BioMed Central, and the Cochrane Library. A total of 16,145 articles were identified. Studies that met the inclusion criteria included systematic reviews and meta-analyses evaluating treatment options for musculoskeletal pain.

1. Opioids

The use of opioids to treat chronic pain has significantly increased over the last few decades. It is estimated that between 5 to 8 million Americans currently use opioids for their chronic pain. Additionally, opioid misuse has escalated dramatically, with prescriptions rising from 76 million in 1991 to 219 million in 2011. The Centers for Disease Control (CDC) has reported a sharp increase in opioid abuse, including a rise in hospital admissions due to addiction to prescribed opioids—from about 40,000 in 2000 to over 160,000 by 2010. In 2015, the United States witnessed 52,404 drug overdose deaths; of these, 20,101 were related to prescription pain relievers, and 12,990 were linked to heroin. Notably, in 2010, one out of every eight deaths among those aged 25 to

34 was related to opioid use. In Georgia, the number of deaths from drug overdoses exceeded those from motor vehicle accidents in 2014. While many patients, providers, and advocates recognize that opioids can manage pain in specific patient groups, the potential for adverse reactions poses a growing concern.

According to the National Institutes of Health, research on the long-term effects of opioid use on pain and functioning is lacking. This pertains to patients who have used opioids daily or nearly daily for two months or more. Observational studies have indicated that patients who use opioids, particularly at higher doses, exhibit lower functional status and quality of life compared to those who do not use opioids or who are on lower doses. Additionally, patients who discontinue opioids during rehabilitation services tend to experience improved function and pain relief. Despite ample research demonstrating the positive effects of opioids on short-term pain, the scarcity of long-term data combined with substantial evidence of adverse effects complicates this controversial issue. Consequently, long-term opioid use may not be the most reliable method for managing chronic pain.

Clinical trials conducted by Xue et al. involving 316 patients have shown that opioid medications do not provide long-term benefits for chronic musculoskeletal pain and are more commonly associated with severe adverse events such as nausea, constipation, hyperalgesia, and drowsiness. These negative effects might impede patients from engaging in more effective management programs. While opioids have been proven to effectively reduce pain in the short term, randomized controlled trials (RCTs) have demonstrated their ineffectiveness for long-term pain relief.

2. Non-steroidal Anti-inflammatory Drugs (NSAIDs)

For many patients and providers, the use of NSAIDs for pain reduction is a common choice. A systematic review assessing the efficacy of NSAIDs on spinal pain evaluated 35 trials. While NSAIDs were found to be effective for short-term spinal pain relief, the results were not clinically significant when compared to placebo groups. It was concluded that an effective long-term analgesic for spinal pain is still needed, as none currently available have been proven effective for prolonged use.

The pain reduction effects of NSAIDs are temporary and may lead to adverse outcomes. For instance, a systematic review by Varas-Lorenzo C et al. indicated that the current use of rofecoxib and diclofenac could increase the risk of ischemic stroke. However, this research focused solely on these two NSAIDs, underscoring the need for further studies to assess other NSAIDs and to determine the doses and durations that heighten the risk of stroke and its subtypes. Overall, the use of NSAIDs for pain reduction has been shown to be ineffective for long-term management, as systematic reviews reveal that they only provide temporary relief.

3. Stretching and Exercises

Stretches and exercises are utilized for various purposes including pain management, injury prevention, and improving range of motion and function. In a 2015 systematic review by Gross et al., 27 trials involving 2,485 analyzed and 3,005 randomized participants were reviewed to assess the effectiveness of exercise in improving pain, disability, function, patient satisfaction, and quality of life for individuals with mechanical neck disorders. The participants included adults suffering from neck pain with or without cervicogenic headache or radiculopathy. The results were mixed: no evidence was found for acute neck pain, moderate quality evidence was found for chronic neck pain and chronic cervicogenic headache, and low quality evidence was found for acute radiculopathy. The review concluded that due to the lack of high-quality evidence, the effectiveness of exercise for treating neck pain remains uncertain.

However, strengthening exercises were noted to be potentially beneficial for chronic neck pain, cervicogenic headache, and radiculopathy, as well as strength and endurance exercises for the cervico-scapulothoracic and shoulder areas.

A 2014 systematic review by Da Silva Filho et al. of 32 studies assessed the effectiveness of stretching for posture correction. The researchers found very little evidence to support the effectiveness of this treatment modality. Additionally, a 2004 systematic review by Thacker et al. of six studies sought to determine if stretching could reduce the risk of sports injuries. The review found no evidence supporting the continuation or discontinuation of stretching before or after exercise to reduce the risk of injury.

In a 2008 systematic review of seven randomized controlled trials, Small et al. found that stretching did not decrease the overall incidence of exercise-related injuries. However, they did observe a reduction in musculotendinous injuries as a result of static stretching.

A systematic review by Gordan and Bloxham analyzed 480 studies, but only 14 met the inclusion criteria regarding the impact of physical activity or exercise interventions on patients with non-specific chronic low back pain (NSCLBP). The study specifically looked at the effects of aerobic exercise, muscular strength and stabilization exercises, and/or flexibility training. The researchers concluded that these exercise programs were beneficial for NSCLBP but did not alleviate acute low back pain, as exercise increased swelling in the affected area.

Another systematic review by Saragiotto et al. examined 2,431 studies, including 29 trials that met the criteria on how motor control exercise (MCE) can aid in the relief of nonspecific low-back pain. The review found very low to moderate evidence that MCE can clinically help chronic low-back pain, low-quality evidence of its clinically important effect compared with exercise plus electrophysical agents, and moderate to high-quality evidence that it offers similar outcomes to manual therapies. Additionally, it found low to moderate quality evidence that MCE provides similar outcomes to other forms of exercise. Given that MCE is not superior to other treatment methods, the choice of exercise for lower-back pain should depend on patient or therapist preferences

In a systematic review by Miller et al., researchers evaluated whether a combination of manual therapy and exercise was more effective than either intervention alone for adults with acute to chronic neck pain, with or without radiculopathy or cervicogenic headache. From 31 different publications and 1,820 citations, 17 trials focused on acute neck pain, five on whiplash-associated disorders, one on degenerative changes, five on cervicogenic headache, and three on neck disorders. The findings indicated that manual therapy alone provided greater short-term pain relief than exercise alone, but no long-term differences were observed across the multiple outcomes for acute/chronic neck pain. Moderate quality evidence supports combining manual therapy and exercise for better pain reduction and improved quality of life over manual therapy alone for chronic neck pain. This approach also showed greater short-term pain reduction compared to traditional care for acute whiplash. However, the reviews suggested that while combining manual therapy and exercise offers better short-term pain relief than either method alone, no long-term effects were noted.

Another systematic review by Chou et al. analyzed 122 trials that assessed the effectiveness of exercise in treating low back pain, including 37 trials focused on exercise. The results revealed no significant difference between exercise therapy and no exercise regarding pain relief. Furthermore, in over 20 head-to-head trials comparing different exercise techniques for acute or chronic back pain, no clear differences were observed. Overall, a vast amount of systematic reviews indicate that stretches and exercises provide little to no long-term pain relief.

4. Massage Therapy

Massage therapy is a commonly used method for reducing pain and relieving muscle tension. A 2015 systematic review by Bervoets et al., which examined 26 randomized trials involving 2,565 participants, found that massage therapy alone was more effective in reducing pain and improving function compared to no treatment. However, it was less effective in reducing pain and improving some musculoskeletal conditions when compared to other active treatments. Another systematic review by Chou et al. analyzed nine trials on massage therapy; one trial reported small improvements on the Roland Morris Disability Questionnaire after massage therapy, but most trials found no significant difference in pain and function outcomes. While most studies noted an increase in efficacy of massage therapy for short-term pain relief, they did not show significant benefits for long-term pain management

Another systematic review by Furlan et al. investigated the effectiveness of massage therapy on low back and neck pain. The study found that subjects with nonspecific acute or sub-acute pain who received massage therapy exhibited significantly reduced pain intensity and disability compared to those receiving no treatment or placebo, both immediately and in the short term after treatment. The review also noted that, compared to no treatment, massage therapy significantly improved pain intensity but not range of motion in subjects with chronic or undetermined duration of nonspecific pain immediately after treatment. While massage therapy has been proven to be more effective in reducing pain compared to no treatment at all, systematic reviews have shown that this method does not offer long-term pain reduction.

5. Acupuncture

Acupuncture is a non-traditional approach to relieving muscle pain; however, its clinical effectiveness remains unclear. A systematic review of 63 randomized controlled trials, which included 6,382 participants by Yuan et al., assessed the effectiveness of acupuncture for musculoskeletal pain. The researchers found that acupuncture reduced pain by about 12 points on the 100mm visual analogue scale, demonstrating only low-quality evidence of its effectiveness. In another systematic review, Madsen et al. analyzed 13 trials involving 3,025 participants, comparing the outcomes among those who received acupuncture, placebo acupuncture, and no acupuncture at all. These treatments spanned from 1 day to 12 weeks and addressed conditions like knee osteoarthritis, tension headaches, migraines, low back pain, fibromyalgia, abdominal scar pain, postoperative pain, and pain during colonoscopy procedures. While there was a moderate difference between the placebo acupuncture and no acupuncture groups, the difference between the acupuncture and placebo acupuncture groups was small. The study concluded that acupuncture's small analgesic effect appears to lack clinical relevance and cannot be clearly distinguished from bias.

Another systematic review of 21 trials by Andrea Furlan assessed the effectiveness of acupuncture compared to no treatment, sham acupuncture, and other therapies for treating chronic low-back pain. The results indicated that while acupuncture appeared more effective than no treatment, it was not more effective than other treatments. Additionally, a separate study by Furlan et al. evaluated acupuncture's effectiveness in treating neck pain, finding inconsistent results between acupuncture and pain medication groups for immediate or short-term post-treatment pain intensity. Acupuncture did not differ significantly from standard mobilization and traction techniques or laser therapy in terms of short-term post-treatment pain intensity or disability. Immediate/short-term post-treatment pain and disability outcomes were better with manipulation than with acupuncture.

Another systematic review by Chou et al. focused on acupuncture for back pain, evaluating 49 trials but only including 11 that addressed acute or subacute back pain. This review found that acupuncture reduced pain intensity more than sham acupuncture with non-penetrating needles for acute low back pain, yet it had no clear effects on function. Overall, these systematic reviews suggest that acupuncture provides only a marginal improvement over placebo, offering short-term pain relief without long-term benefits.

6. Steroid Injections

Steroid injections, also known as corticosteroid injections, are medical treatments used to temporarily reduce inflammation and alleviate pain in various parts of the body. These injections typically contain a corticosteroid medication and sometimes a local anesthetic. They are frequently used to treat a range of conditions, including joint pain, arthritis, sciatica, and inflammatory skin conditions. Godwin et al.'s systematic review with meta-analysis examined five randomized controlled trials involving 312 patients. They concluded that corticosteroid injections result in clinically and statistically significant reductions in osteoarthritic knee pain one week after injection. The beneficial effects could last for three to four weeks, but are unlikely to continue beyond that.

Gazendam et al.'s systematic review and meta-analysis of randomized controlled trials investigated whether intra-articular (hip) saline injections are as effective as corticosteroids, platelet-rich plasma, and hyaluronic acid for managing hip osteoarthritis pain. They evaluated eleven randomized controlled trials comprising 1,353 patients. They found that none of the hip injections demonstrated significant improvement in function scores when compared with saline hip injections at 2–4 months (9 trials, 968 patients) or 6 months (9 trials, 995 patients).

The University of South Australia published a systematic review of the literature titled "The Effectiveness of Knee Injection of Steroid With or Without Local Anesthetic." This study found that 13 systematic reviews met the inclusion criteria for this review. They concluded, "The evidence indicates that the addition of intra-articular steroids in conjunction with a 12-week exercise program offers no additional benefit compared to the exercise program alone in patients with osteoarthritis."

Guermazi et al.'s review "Intra-articular corticosteroids (IACS) injections for osteoarthritis – harmful or helpful?" the researches concludes" IACS injection has not clearly demonstrated long-term efficacy for treating joint pains in knee or hip osteoarthritis. IACS injection is not totally safe, given the documented adverse joint events in the literature"

7. Dry Needle

Dry needling is used for managing various neuromusculoskeletal pain syndromes by targeting muscles, ligaments, tendons, scar tissue, subcutaneous fascia, peripheral nerves, and neurovascular bundles. It is defined as the insertion of a solid needle through the skin without introducing any drugs, aiming to stimulate trigger points and connective tissue to manage neuro-musculoskeletal pain.

In a systematic review, Morihisa et al. assessed the effectiveness of dry needling for alleviating symptoms associated with muscular trigger points. After screening

2,232 potential studies, only six met the inclusion criteria. The review concluded that dry needling effectively reduces pain associated with lower quarter trigger points in the short term. However, it does not significantly impact function, quality of life, depression, range of motion, or strength.

A systematic review by Gattie et al., which included 13 studies and 723 participants, assessed the effectiveness of dry needling for musculoskeletal conditions over a 12-week follow-up period. The evidence, ranging from low to moderate quality, suggests that dry needling performed by physical therapists is more effective than no treatment, sham dry needling, and other treatments in reducing pain and improving pressure pain threshold. Additionally, a small but significant effect was observed in improving functional outcomes compared to no treatment or sham needling. However, there is currently a lack of evidence supporting the long-term benefits of dry needling.

In another systematic review, Matthew Cotchett et al. evaluated the effectiveness of dry needling and/or injections for myofascial trigger points associated with plantar heel pain. Out of 342 studies identified, only three quasi-experimental studies met the inclusion criteria. Plantar heel pain is one of the most common musculoskeletal pathologies of the foot, estimated to affect 10% of the population at some point in their lives. The review utilized a narrative synthesis due to the poor methodological quality and heterogeneous nature of the studies, concluding that there is limited evidence supporting the effectiveness of dry needling and/or injections for plantar heel pain.

A literature review by Dunning et al. suggests that while several studies have shown immediate or short-term improvements in pain and/or disability by targeting muscular trigger points with dry needling, there are no high-quality long-term trials that support this technique. Overall, dry needling has been beneficial for reducing pain in the short term, but evidence supporting its long-term effectiveness is lacking.

Similarly, a systematic review of 15 studies by Espejo-Antunez et al. evaluated the effectiveness of dry needle treatment for myofascial trigger points compared to other interventions such as oral drugs, acupuncture, and placebo. Although the evidence suggests that dry needling may positively affect pain and mobility in the short term compared to placebo, no studies have demonstrated long-term effects. Multiple systematic reviews confirm that while dry needling is effective in temporarily reducing pain, there is insufficient evidence to conclude that this method provides long-term pain relief.

8. Trigger Point Injection

Myofascial trigger point pain is defined as pain originating from one or more myofascial trigger points—hyper-irritable spots in skeletal muscle associated with hypersensitive palpable nodules in taut bands. A systematic review by Cummings and White evaluated the effectiveness of trigger point injection therapy for myofascial pain, including a total of 23 randomized controlled trials that tested needle therapy to relieve this condition. The review found that while needling was effective, the positive effects were more likely attributed to the placebo effect of the needle rather than the injected drug, showing no significant pain improvement between direct needling and placebo.

Scott et al. assessed the effectiveness of trigger point injections for chronic non-malignant musculoskeletal pain in their systematic review. This study included participants whose pain lasted more than three months and incorporated 15 randomized controlled trials. The researchers found no conclusive evidence supporting the effectiveness or ineffectiveness of trigger point injections. Additionally, a systematic review by Matthew Cotchett et al. examined the effectiveness of dry needling and/or injections at myofascial trigger points associated with plantar heel pain. Out of 342 studies identified, only three quasi-experimental studies met the inclusion criteria. The review indicates limited evidence supporting the effectiveness of these treatments for plantar heel pain, largely due to the poor quality and heterogeneous nature of the studies included. Overall, the systematic reviews assessed suggest a lack of evidence supporting the long-term effectiveness of trigger point injection therapy for pain relief.

9. Therapeutic Ultrasound

Therapeutic ultrasound is a treatment modality commonly used by physical therapists and other healthcare professionals to manage pain. A systematic review by Aiyer et al. investigated the effect of ultrasound on chronic joint pain management. The review included 8 trials for the knee and 7 trials for the shoulder that met the inclusion criteria of the study. The researchers concluded, "As a monotherapy, ultrasound treatment may not have a significant impact on functional improvement."

10. Electrical Stimulation

Electrical stimulation for pain management commonly refers to Transcutaneous Electrical Nerve Stimulation (TENS). This method is used to manage pain by delivering electrical signals to the nervous system. Deng et al.'s systematic review titled "Electrical Stimulation Therapy for Patients with Neurogenic Bowel Dysfunction After Spinal Cord Injury" included 11 clinical studies with a total of 298 participants who met the inclusion criteria. They concluded, "There was currently not enough evidence to support the use of electrical stimulation to improve the clinical symptoms of those patients."

11. Platelet-Rich Plasma (PRP)

Platelet-rich plasma (PRP) is a concentrated form of plasma, one of the components of blood, that contains a high level of platelets. These platelets are crucial for blood clotting and are rich in growth factors, which are important for healing injuries. PRP is produced by taking a sample of blood from the patient, then processing it in a centrifuge to concentrate the platelets before reinjecting it into the affected area.

Lui et al.'s systematic review and meta-analysis titled "Nonoperative Platelet-Rich Plasma Shoulder Injections for Rotator Cuff Pathology" included six studies that met the systematic review criteria. They concluded, "There is a limited quantity of high-quality studies that assess the efficacy of nonoperative PRP shoulder injections for pain and range of motion (ROM). The systematic review of PRP injections did not demonstrate an improvement in pain or ROM compared to physical therapy."

Gazendam et al.'s systematic review and meta-analysis of randomized controlled trials investigated whether intra-articular (hip) saline injections are as effective as corticosteroids, platelet-rich plasma, and hyaluronic acid for managing hip osteoarthritis pain. They evaluated eleven randomized controlled trials comprising 1,353 patients. They found that "None of the hip injections demonstrated significant improvement in function scores when compared with saline hip injections at 2–4 months (9 trials, 968 patients) or 6 months (9 trials, 995 patients)".

12. Manual Therapy - Soft Tissue Mobilization

Manual therapy appears to offer short-term benefits in pain reduction. A 2010 systematic review by Miller et al., which examined 17 controlled randomized trials on the efficacy of exercise and manual therapy for neck pain, found no long-term differences in outcomes for (sub)acute or chronic neck pain, with or without cervicogenic headaches.

Another review by Penas et al. assessed the effectiveness of manual therapy in treating myofascial trigger points (MTrP). The results did not provide rigorous evidence that manual therapies are more effective than placebo in treating MTrP. Although manual therapy can reduce pain and improve range of motion in the short term, these systematic reviews suggest that there is a lack of evidence supporting its long-term benefits.

13. Instrument Assisted Soft Tissue Mobilization (IASTM)

Specially designed instruments are used by physical therapists, occupational therapists, and chiropractors to address soft tissue adhesions. A systematic review of seven randomized controlled trials by Cheatham et al. examined the efficacy of Instrument Assisted Soft Tissue Mobilization (IASTM). The review found insufficient evidence to support the benefit of IASTM for treating musculoskeletal conditions, although some evidence suggested it could increase joint range of motion in the short term. While the use of such instruments may temporarily enhance range of motion, this systematic review indicates a lack of evidence for any long-term effects.

14. Myofascial Release

Self-myofascial release (SMFR) is a popular method used to improve myofascial mobility. Common tools employed in this method include foam rolls and roller massages. A systematic review by Cheatham et al. analyzed 14 articles that met the inclusion criteria, involving 260 healthy subjects (179 males and 81 females), with an average age of 19.6 years, ranging from 15 to 34 years old. The studies examined the effects of using a foam roller on hip, knee, and ankle range of motion (ROM), as well as on foam rolling sit and reach exercises. Five studies specifically used roller massages to assess ankle, knee, and hip ROM, and roller massage sit and reach. The researchers found that SMFR, whether with a foam roller or roller massage, can have short-term effects on increasing joint ROM without adversely affecting muscle performance. Additionally, they noted that SMFR could help mitigate decrements in muscle performance and delayed onset muscle soreness following intense exercise. However, they also emphasized that there is currently not enough high-quality evidence to draw firm conclusions.

In a systematic review by [Author(s)] et al., researchers assessed studies on the acute and chronic clinical effects of SMFR. They concluded that SMFR increases flexibility, reduces muscle soreness, and does not hinder athletic performance. The review also found that SMFR could improve arterial function, vascular endothelial function, and increase parasympathetic nervous system activity, all of which may be beneficial in recovery. However, the evidence is conflicting regarding whether SMFR can improve flexibility over the long term.
The systematic review by Ajimsha et al., which included 19 randomized controlled trials, assessed the effectiveness of myofascial release. The researchers concluded that myofascial release could be useful alone or in

conjunction with other therapies, and that some treatment effects appeared to be retained. However, further examination revealed that 11 of the 19 reviews identified limitations due to the lack of follow-up or reliance solely on immediate follow-up measurements, complicating the assessment of long-term effects.

Additionally, one study that supported long-term effectiveness included myofascial release as part of a multimodal treatment, aligning more with the biopsychosocial model. Given the insufficient follow-up in many studies, the claim that treatment effects are sustained may not be well-supported. While myofascial release has been shown to effectively increase range of motion and reduce pain in the short term without hindering performance, numerous reviews indicate that myofascial release alone does not provide long-term benefits.

15. Joint Manipulation - Joint Mobilization

Joint mobilization is used to restore decreased mobility, though its effectiveness may not be as robust as commonly perceived. A systematic review by Rubinstein et al. examined the effectiveness of spinal manipulation therapy for chronic lower back pain, analyzing 26 randomized controlled trials with 6,070 participants. The evidence showed no significant difference between spinal manipulation therapy and other interventions.

Another systematic review by Young et al., which included five studies, assessed the effectiveness of thoracic manipulation for mechanical neck pain. The researchers found no definitive evidence supporting the efficacy of thoracic manipulation.A study by Canter and Ernst reviewed the effectiveness of spinal manipulation across multiple pain regions, including back and neck pain, involving 16 trials. Their findings indicated that spinal manipulation was ineffective for all evaluated forms of pain.

Lastly, a systematic review by Furlan et al. focused on the effectiveness of joint manipulation and mobilization for low back and neck pain. This review included comparisons of manipulation with placebo, massage, and physiotherapy concerning post-treatment pain, medication intake, disability, and back flexibility, yielding inconsistent results. Specifically, the studies found no significant difference in pain intensity and range of motion between subjects who received mobilization and those who received placebo immediately or in the short term after treatment.

A systematic review by Chou et al. evaluated the effectiveness of spinal manipulation for low back pain. Although 61 trials were initially identified, only 19 met the inclusion criteria and were included in the review. The results indicated that spinal manipulation had small, statistically nonsignificant effects on pain at 1 month compared to sham manipulation, and found no differences in pain relief at 1 week between spinal manipulation and treatments considered inactive.

A 2009 systematic review by Vernon and Schneider examined the effectiveness of manipulation for treating myofascial trigger points (MTrP). The review found moderately strong evidence that supports the use of manipulation and ischemic pressure for immediate pain relief at MTrPs, but only limited evidence for long-term pain relief. Additionally, limited evidence supports the use of electrical muscle stimulation, high-voltage galvanic stimulation, interferential current, and frequency-modulated neural stimulation in treating MTrPs and myofascial pain syndrome, with weak evidence for ultrasound therapy. Based on these systematic reviews, spinal manipulation does not appear to be an effective treatment for various types of pain, including back pain.

16. Manual Therapy and Exercise

Therapeutic exercise and orthopedic manual therapy are the most commonly used treatment methods for impingement syndrome. A systematic review by Desmeules et al. evaluated the effectiveness of these treatments for impingement syndrome, including conditions like rotator cuff tendinitis and bursitis. The review included randomized controlled trials that featured therapeutic exercise or manual therapy as interventions. Out of the studies considered, seven met the inclusion criteria, and four of these suggested some benefits of manual therapy or therapeutic exercise compared to other treatments such as acromioplasty, placebo, or no intervention. However, the evidence supporting the efficacy of these methods for treating impingement syndrome is limited.

In another systematic review by Miller et al., researchers aimed to determine whether combining manual therapy and exercise was more effective than either method alone for treating adults with acute to chronic neck pain, with or without radiculopathy or cervicogenic headache. This review included 17 trials from 31 different publications, which encompassed 1,820 citations. The studies addressed acute neck pain (17 trials), whiplash-associated disorders (5 trials), degenerative changes (1 trial), cervicogenic headache (5 trials), and other neck disorders (3 trials). The findings indicated that manual therapy alone provided greater short-term pain relief than exercise alone, but no long-term differences were observed in the multiple outcomes for acute or chronic neck pain.

Moderate quality evidence supports the combination of manual therapy and exercise over manual therapy alone for reducing pain and improving quality of life in cases of chronic neck pain. This combination also provided greater short-term pain reduction compared to traditional care for acute whiplash. The review concluded that while the combination of manual therapy and exercise offers more effective short-term pain relief than either treatment alone, there is no evidence of long-term benefits from these treatments.

17. Kinesio Taping

Kinesio Taping is a therapeutic technique designed to support fascia, muscles, and joints without restricting motion. It is theorized to improve lymphatic and blood circulation, thereby reducing pain, inflammation, and recovery times. A systematic review by Borchers et al., which examined six studies on the efficacy of Kinesio Taping for musculoskeletal injuries, found insufficient evidence to support or refute its effectiveness in preventing injury, reducing non-injury related inflammation and pain, or decreasing recovery times. The reviews indicate a lack of conclusive evidence regarding the effectiveness of Kinesio Tape in pain management.

18. Active Release Technique (ART)

Active Release Technique is a manual therapy aimed at restoring function in soft tissues by removing scar tissue that may lead to stiffness, pain, mechanical dysfunctions, and muscle weaknesses. There is limited research on ART, with only one randomized study among several pilot studies. This trial, conducted by Kim et al., involved 24 subjects with neck pain lasting more than three months. It compared the effectiveness of ART and joint mobilization in increasing range of motion. The results showed that both treatments improved chronic neck pain, but ART yielded greater improvements in cases involving soft tissue injuries. However, the small sample size and limited data on patient functional activities make it difficult to conclusively determine its clinical effectiveness. Although ART showed short-term effectiveness, further studies are necessary to assess its long-term impacts and effects on patient function.

19. Strain Counterstrain Technique (SCS)

Strain Counterstrain is a technique that uses passive positioning to alleviate pain from tender point palpations and associated dysfunctions. A systematic review by Wong et al. included randomized controlled trials that compared pain levels using a visual analog scale after isolated strain counterstrain treatment versus control conditions. The meta-analysis revealed low-quality evidence suggesting that strain counterstrain may reduce tender point palpation pain. However, there is no evidence supporting its effectiveness in long-term treatment of tender point pain.

20. Craniosacral Therapy

Craniosacral Therapy focuses on releasing restrictions around the spinal cord and brain to restore body function. A systematic review by Jakel and Von Hauenschild evaluated the clinical benefits of craniosacral therapy using studies that involved only this therapy as a treatment. The review included 7 studies: 3 randomized controlled trials and 4 observational studies. These studies highlighted a shortage of research on craniosacral therapy across various clinical pathologies. Although feasible in randomized control trials and potentially valuable for clinical decision-making, the methodological quality of existing studies necessitates further research.

Another systematic review by Green et al. aimed to assess the biological plausibility, reliability, and clinical effectiveness of craniosacral therapy. They analyzed 33 studies, 7 of which provided data on its effectiveness. The review concluded that there is insufficient evidence to consider craniosacral therapy clinically effective due to the low quality of the evidence and inadequate research protocols. Current research methods have not yet conclusively evaluated the effectiveness of this therapy.

21. McKenzie Method

The McKenzie method, a popular approach for managing spinal pain, tailors treatment to individual patient conditions. A systematic review by Clare et al. examined the efficacy of McKenzie therapy for spinal pain, analyzing 24 studies, including 6 randomized trials. The review found that McKenzie therapy resulted in a significant short-term pain reduction, averaging 8.6 points on a 100-point scale, and showed benefits comparable to an exercise program in one cervical trial. However, long-term effects remain under-researched.

In another systematic review by Machado et al., 11 randomized trials evaluated the McKenzie method for low back pain. At a one-week follow-up, there was a modest pain reduction of -4.16 points and a disability reduction of -5.22 points compared with passive therapy for acute lower back pain. At a 12-week follow-up, when compared with 'stay active' advice, the reduction in disability favored the advice. The review suggested that while the McKenzie method is more effective than passive therapy, the differences are not clinically significant. Evidence for its use in chronic low back pain is limited.

Summary

Based on an overwhelming number of studies, the following treatments have demonstrated either short-term pain reduction or no pain reduction for musculoskeletal pain. In some cases, the placebo effect performed better than the biomedical model due to the severe adverse effects of the biomedical model treatments. Here is the list of ineffective treatments for chronic pain:

1. Opioids
2. Non-steroidal Anti-inflammatory Drugs (NSAIDs)
3. Stretching and Exercises
4. Massage Therapy
5. Acupuncture
6. Steroid injections
7. Trigger Point Injection
8. Dry Needle
9. Therapeutic Ultrasound
10. Electrical Stimulation
11. Platelet-Rich Plasma (PRP)
12. Manual Therapy - Soft Tissue Mobilization
13. Instrument Assisted Soft Tissue Mobilization (IASTM)
14. Myofascial Release
15. Joint Manipulation - Joint Mobilization
16. Manual Therapy and Exercise
17. Kinesio Taping
18. Active Release Technique (ART)
19. Strain Counterstrain Technique (SCS)
20. Craniosacral Therapy
21. McKenzie Method

In the following chapter, we will explore the biopsychosocial (BPS) model and present studies demonstrating its efficacy.

The Biopsychosocial Model: A Paradigm Shift in Health Care

The BPS Model

Before explaining the biopsychosocial (BPS) model, it's important to understand what constitutes a disease. We also need to familiarize ourselves with the biomedical model (commonly referred to as Western medicine). This knowledge will provide a foundation for appreciating the BPS approach.

What is Disease?

The definition of disease from Merriam-Webster dictionary is "a condition of the living animal or plant body or of one of its parts that impairs normal functioning and is typically manifested by distinguishing signs and symptoms." Disease is basically a condition that consists of signs and symptoms that are abnormal to the human body. This definition does not help us to understand or treat the root cause of the problem. It focuses on signs and symptoms and does not help healthcare providers to answer the question of why patients are experiencing the condition and how to treat the root cause of the issue.

What is the Biomedical Model?

The biomedical model, which is also known as Western medicine or allopathic medicine, focuses on pathophysiology and other biological approaches to disease. Essentially, the biomedical model emphasizes the biological effects of disease and the treatment focuses on the signs and symptoms of the condition. This was the main issue I faced after my second cancer treatment: I could not receive the medical help to address the root cause of my fatigue, pain, and migraines. The doctors kept recommending pain and migraine medication without trying to figure out why I had these issues. That led me to search for an answer and stumble upon the BPS model in research literature.

What is Idiopathic?

'Idiopathic' is a term used in medicine to describe a condition or disease that arises spontaneously or for which the cause is unknown. It is derived from the Greek words 'idios,' meaning 'one's own,' and 'pathos,' meaning 'suffering.' When a condition is labeled idiopathic, it means that despite thorough investigation, no specific cause or origin can be identified. This term is often used in the context of idiopathic diseases or conditions, such as idiopathic pulmonary fibrosis, idiopathic epilepsy, fibromyalgia, chronic fatigue syndrome, stroke, irritable bowel syndrome, idiopathic hypertension, Parkinson's disease, peripheral neuropathy, ulcerative colitis, scoliosis, juvenile arthritis, etc. There are many diseases in the biomedical model that are considered to be of idiopathic origin. This leads to an inability to treat the root cause of the problem, resulting in a focus on managing symptoms.

Example of Biomedical Treatment Model

The biomedical model is successful in saving people's lives by quickly lowering extremely high blood pressure to prevent strokes or heart attacks. It is also effective for tumor removal, gunshot wound treatment, Coronary Artery Bypass Grafting (CABG) surgery, Aortic Aneurysm Repair, Craniotomy for Stroke, Hemorrhage Control, Appendectomy, and other similar procedures. The biomedical model is very effective in addressing life-threatening conditions and injuries to save lives. However, it has failed to address chronic conditions.

I was labeled as a fibromyalgia, chronic fatigue, and irritable bowel syndrome (IBS) patient. These are idiopathic diseases based on the biomedical model, and I met many others with the same diagnosis. However, after studying the BPS model and implementing proper nutrition evaluation and treatment, I was able to resolve my conditions. This indicates that nutrition, vitamin, mineral, and hormonal imbalances may lead to idiopathic diseases such as fibromyalgia, chronic fatigue, and IBS.

Nutrition Education: A Missing Component in Medical Schools

One of the main problems I faced when I had chronic fatigue and pain was that doctors did not evaluate my malnutrition, which was the underlying issue. Later, after talking to many doctors, I noticed that none of them had proper nutrition education in medical school. It makes sense now—if you do not have the proper education, you cannot evaluate it. This surprised me; even in physical therapy school, we did not have enough nutrition education. That is what led several medical doctors to come and ask me what the best diet is and what to eat to stay healthy.

The lack of nutrition education in medical school is similar to a mechanic attending mechanic school but not receiving any education in the curriculum about the different types of car fluids or the specific gas needed for different car parts or brands. Many diseases have a strong relation to malnutrition, including obesity, infections, type II diabetes, celiac disease, Crohn's disease, cardiovascular diseases, kwashiorkor, marasmus, rickets, scurvy, beriberi, pellagra, anemia, osteoporosis, night blindness, goiter, hypocalcemia, hypomagnesemia, protein-energy malnutrition (PEM), zinc deficiency, copper deficiency, vitamin K deficiency, vitamin E deficiency, folate deficiency, vitamin B6 deficiency, and omega-3 fatty acid deficiency. If doctors do not know how to perform a nutrition evaluation, how can they provide proper treatment for patients with malnutrition?

Case Study 1: Chronic Pain, Fatigue, and Headaches

For my chronic pain, fatigue, and headaches, doctors recommended pain medication, muscle relaxers, and Gabapentin. Because I had constipation, a stool softener was recommended. Due to severe stress from my pain, which caused increased blood pressure, medication to lower blood pressure was also suggested. This is an example of the biomedical model that addresses the disease's signs and symptoms. I noticed that all these medications were properly prescribed to address the symptoms, but I had severe side effects. This made me question why I was doing this, as I was not receiving treatment that addressed the root cause of the problem.

Case Study 2: Frequent Sickness

During the time I had chronic fatigue, joint pain, and migraines, I used to get very sick frequently. I remember one visit to the doctor for a cold episode. The doctor asked about my symptoms, so I explained that I had a cough,

congestion, fatigue, sore throat, headache, runny nose, and body aches. The doctor prescribed four different medications to address the symptoms: pain medication, cough suppressants, decongestants, and antihistamines.
Based on the biomedical model, the doctor properly addressed the disease symptoms. The main problem is that none of the medications addressed the root cause of the issue. The root cause was a very weak immune system due to malnutrition and severe vitamin, mineral, and hormonal imbalances. I discovered these imbalances later after studying nutrition and was able to stay healthy without being frequently sick.

What is the Biopsychosocial (BPS)?

The BPS model is a treatment option that assesses and integrates the biological, psychological, and social factors in understanding health, illness, and disease. It is a holistic approach that looks at the health problem from all angles to understand and address it from all problematic sides. It is like looking at the problem from three-dimensional aspects. In contrast, the biomedical model looks at diseases from the biological effects of signs and symptoms and hyper-focuses on the symptoms instead of looking at all aspects of the problem.

The BPS model is a systematic approach that considers biological, psychological, and social factors and their complex interactions in understanding health, illness, and implementing healthcare treatment.

Components of the Biopsychosocial Model:

1. **Biological Element:** These include genetic predispositions, physical health, brain chemistry, injuries, and other conditions that can affect health physically. It is the physical part of the illness.
2. **Psychological Element:** This aspect covers a range of influences such as mood, personality, behavior, stress response, and coping mechanisms that can impact health outcomes.

3. **Social Element:** Social determinants of health, such as socioeconomic status, culture, poverty, technology, access to healthcare, and social support systems, significantly influence an individual's health status.

History of Biopsychosocial

In 1977, American pathologist and psychiatrist Dr. George Engel (1913-1999) developed the BPS model and published his paper titled 'The Need for a New Medical Model: A Challenge for Biomedicine' in the journal Science.

The following section presents detailed research study findings. If you do not like to read <u>dry scientific information</u>, you can skip to the 'Challenges of Implementing the Biopsychosocial Model' section.

Biopsychosocial Research

1. Turk and Okifuji Literature Review

Turk and Okifuji, in their literature review, argue that no specific surgical procedures, pharmacological agents, or physical treatment methods have shown long-term effectiveness in treating chronic pain. They emphasize that pain not only affects individuals physically but also contributes to negative emotional states. Pain encompasses psychological and environmental factors in addition to physical injury. The researchers highlight the significant advancements in the development of multidisciplinary, holistic treatment approaches. Despite third-party payers often favoring surgery, they note that most patients at multidisciplinary pain clinics have undergone unsuccessful surgeries, suggesting that multidisciplinary clinics could be a more cost-effective alternative. They also point out that over 60% of individuals in these clinics have multiple psychological impairments, underscoring the importance of a holistic approach. The research suggests that multidisciplinary pain clinics achieve a 20-30% reduction in pain, which either remains stable or continues to decrease.

2. Systematic Review by Tzenalis et al.

In a systematic review by Tzenalis et al., researchers evaluated 23 randomized controlled trials to compare the biopsychosocial model against other treatment methods, used either together or individually. This model incorporated medical, educational, cognitive-behavioral therapy, relaxation, biofeedback, and social therapy components. The study included participants aged 18 to 75 who had chronic pain lasting more than 12 weeks. The review concluded that cognitive-behavioral rehabilitation, a key component of the biopsychosocial model, provides long-term pain relief.

3. Systematic Review by Kamper et al.

Kamper et al. conducted a systematic review to assess the long-term effectiveness of multidisciplinary treatment approaches for individuals with chronic lower back pain, many of whom had previously tried other treatments unsuccessfully. This review included 41 trials, involving 6,858 participants, with 16 trials comparing usual care to multidisciplinary approaches and 19 comparing these approaches to physical treatment methods. The findings indicated moderate quality evidence of the superior effectiveness of the multidisciplinary approach compared to usual care and demonstrated that multidisciplinary rehabilitation programs significantly improved outcomes concerning long-term pain and disability when compared to usual care (moderate quality evidence) or physical treatments (low quality evidence).

4. Systematic Review by Guzmán et al.

Guzmán et al. conducted a systematic review to assess the effectiveness of a biopsychosocial treatment approach for individuals suffering from chronic low back pain. This review included randomized controlled trials involving 1,964 participants who had experienced low back pain for at least three months. The study included 10 trials where the biopsychosocial method was compared to a control group, which did not receive a multidisciplinary treatment approach. The results strongly suggest that the biopsychosocial approach was more effective in improving functionality compared to non-multidisciplinary treatments, with moderate evidence supporting its superior effectiveness in pain management.

5. Systematic Review by Karjalainen et al.

Karjalainen et al. aimed to evaluate the effectiveness of multidisciplinary biopsychosocial rehabilitation for subacute low back pain among adults. Out of 1,808 references, only two relevant studies were included. The review found moderate evidence that multidisciplinary rehabilitation helps patients return to work faster and reduces sick leave.

6. Systematic Review by Ospina and Harstall

Ospina and Harstall's systematic review focused on evaluating the effectiveness of multidisciplinary pain programs for chronic pain. Out of 13 systematic reviews considered relevant, only five met the inclusion criteria. The chosen review included 65 controlled and non-controlled trials, supporting the effectiveness of intensive multidisciplinary pain programs in terms of functional improvement and pain reduction.

7. Systematic Review by Van Geen et al.

Van Geen et al. reviewed the long-term effect of multidisciplinary back training on work participation among patients with chronic low back pain. They identified 10 studies that met the inclusion criteria, half of which were of low methodological quality. The five high-quality studies each reported positive effects on at least one of four measured outcomes. The review concluded that multidisciplinary back training positively impacts work participation in the long term.

Challenges of Implementing the Biopsychosocial Model

The BPS Model

Implementing the BPS model in clinical practice presents several challenges, despite its comprehensive approach to understanding patient health by integrating biological, psychological, and social factors. Here are some key challenges:

1. **Complexity and Time-Consumption:** The BPS model requires a thorough assessment of not just the physical symptoms but also the psychological and social backgrounds of patients. This holistic approach can be time-consuming and complex, making it difficult for healthcare providers who are often under time constraints.

2. **Training and Education**: Many healthcare professionals are traditionally trained in a biomedical model that focuses on physical aspects of illness. Adapting to the BPS model requires additional training and education to understand and integrate psychological and social dimensions effectively.

3. **Interdisciplinary Collaboration**: The BPS model requires collaboration across various specialties, such as psychology, physical therapy, nutrition, social work, and general medicine. Organizing and maintaining such interdisciplinary teams can be logistically challenging and resource-intensive.

4. **Resource Availability**: Implementing the BPS model often requires more resources than traditional methods, including more time per patient and additional personnel. In many healthcare settings, especially those with limited resources, this can be a significant barrier.

5. **Cultural Barriers**: The acceptance and integration of the BPS model can vary culturally. Some cultures may emphasize medical treatments over psychological or social interventions, or there may be stigma associated with acknowledging psychological aspects of illness.

6. **Insurance and Funding**: Healthcare reimbursement systems are often structured around specific procedures in the biomedical model rather than holistic care approaches. Providers may find it challenging to obtain compensation for interventions that address psychological and social components of health.

7. **Patient Acceptance**: Patients accustomed to the biomedical model may expect quick, tangible solutions like medications or surgery and may be less open to approaches that involve in-depth discussions about their lifestyle, nutrition, behavior modification, mental health, or social circumstances.

The Solution

Part of the solution involves learning the BPS model and implementing the aspects that can be done at home, which are presented in this book. This book provides guidance on how to implement several aspects of the BPS model at home. However, some parts of the model require proper evaluation by a healthcare provider who is well-trained in the BPS.

Part of my frustration as a healthcare provider attempting to learn the BPS model was that I couldn't find a single course that covered the entire model comprehensively. Instead, I had to enroll in several different courses, studying each component of the BPS model individually to implement it on myself. This experience led me to realize the need to create a comprehensive course for healthcare providers. This course would enable them to learn the entire model without having to take six to eight different courses from various institutes to implement the model effectively on their patients.

I realized that the BPS model can be implemented by a single healthcare provider instead of five to seven different providers, so I reinvented the model and called it ASTR treatment. Therefore, I have developed courses to enable healthcare providers to do just that.

Advantages of Implementing the Biopsychosocial Model by a Single Healthcare Provider

When the BPS model is implemented by a single healthcare provider, it can offer several significant benefits:

1. **Reduced Healthcare Costs**: Consolidating multiple specialists' roles into a single provider can reduce costs associated with multiple consultations, tests, and treatments often repeated across providers.
2. **Streamlined Care**: Patients can avoid the inconvenience and time consumption of visiting multiple specialists. This streamlined approach

also speeds up the treatment process, as it reduces the waiting times associated with referrals and scheduling with various specialists.

3. **Improved Outcomes**: A single provider is likely to have a more comprehensive understanding of the patient's overall health situation, as they monitor all aspects of the patient's care. This holistic view helps in making more informed decisions, minimizing the risks of miscommunication or conflicting treatments that can occur between multiple providers.

4. **Enhanced Patient Experience**: Patients may feel more at ease and understood when they build a relationship with one provider who addresses all their needs—physical, psychological, and social. This can lead to better compliance with treatment protocols and increased satisfaction with the care received.

5. **Comprehensive Health Management**: By addressing a wide range of factors such as nutrition, ergonomics, behavior modification, stress management, exercises, and physiological imbalances all at once, the provider can more effectively identify and treat the interrelated causes of health issues. This approach leads to more effective and lasting solutions.

6. **Increased Provider Satisfaction**: Providers may find it rewarding to see the full impact of their care across the various aspects of a patient's health. This can enhance job satisfaction and professional fulfillment.

Implementing the BPS model in this manner enables a more personalized, efficient, and effective healthcare experience for both patients and providers. All case studies presented in this book demonstrate that the BPS model can be implemented by a single healthcare provider.

Summary

Overwhelming research studies have confirmed the efficacy of the BPS model in relieving chronic pain, improving quality of life, and transitioning patients back to normal activities. It is more cost-effective and time-efficient when the BPS model is provided by a single healthcare provider. This approach not only improves patient outcomes and experiences but also increases job satisfaction among healthcare providers.

Navigating The Healing Journey: How Your Body Recovers Naturally

Normal Healing Cycle

Inflammation

Increased Temperature
Loss of Function
Redness
Swelling
Pain

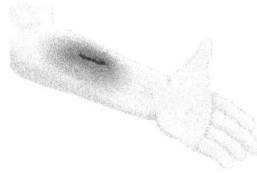

Proliferation

Fibrosis (Scar Tissue)
Fascia Restriction
Muscle Spasm
Trigger Points

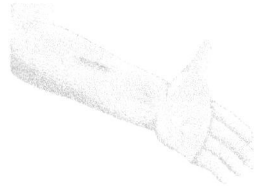

Maturation

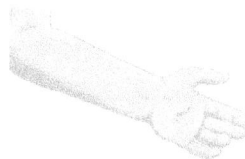

ASTR

Chronic pain impacts a large portion of the population and can be severely disabling, limiting individuals from engaging in everyday activities like work. According to the National Institute of Health, approximately 100 million Americans suffer from chronic pain, with about 25% of these individuals experiencing a reduced quality of life and significant restrictions in their activities due to moderate to severe pain. In 2010, the prevalence of chronic pain (lasting more than three months) was estimated at 30.7% for U.S. adults, with a higher prevalence in females compared to males.

Understanding the normal body healing cycle helps in evaluating current treatments and choosing the appropriate ones to address the root cause of chronic pain. This knowledge guides us in selecting treatments that effectively target the underlying issue.

The normal healing cycle consists of three stages, which can be illustrated using an external paper cut to visualize what happens internally in the body. See the image below for more details. The first stage is inflammation, characterized by swelling, redness, pain, and increased blood flow to the affected area. The second stage involves the formation of fibrosis, also known as scar tissue, which fills the wound to prevent it from remaining open and susceptible to infection. During this stage, the injured site may also experience fascial restrictions and muscle spasms. This highlights the essential role of scar tissue in our protection and survival.

The third stage of the healing cycle involves the breakdown of fibrotic tissue. Ideally, in a perfect world with perfect bodies, the body would autonomously break down this fibrotic tissue over a period of days, weeks, or months, depending on the severity of the injury. However, we do not live in a perfect world. As we age, our body's ability to break down scar tissue decreases significantly.

This healing process also occurs internally when our bodies experience injuries from accidents, surgeries, trauma, poor posture, or stress. Below, the normal muscle healing process after injury is described in more depth, outlining a complex sequence that can be divided into several overlapping phases. The duration of each phase can vary depending on the severity of the injury and the individual's overall health. In chronic conditions, the injured area may not progress through all three stages, instead getting stuck between the inflammation and proliferation stages. Here is a breakdown of the normal muscle healing cycle:

Destruction Stage (Injury Initiation)

This initial phase begins immediately after injury and is characterized by the disruption of muscle fibers and blood vessels, leading to the formation of a hematoma (a localized collection of blood outside of blood vessels). The hematoma serves to contain the damage and forms a scaffold for incoming inflammatory cells.

1. Inflammatory Stage

This phase starts within hours after the injury and can last for several days. It involves the following key processes:

- **Inflammation**: In response to injury, inflammatory cells such as neutrophils and macrophages infiltrate the site. They remove debris, damaged cells, and pathogens. This phase is associated with the classic signs of inflammation: redness, heat, swelling, and pain.
- **Release of Cytokines**: Inflammatory cells release cytokines and growth factors that are crucial for healing and recruiting more reparative cells to the injury site.

2. Proliferation Stage

During this phase, the focus shifts from clearing out the debris to rebuilding muscle tissue, and typically lasts from several days to a couple of weeks:

- **Myogenesis**: This is the formation of new muscle fibers through the activation, differentiation, and fusion of myoblasts (muscle progenitor cells).
- **Fibroblast Proliferation**: Fibroblasts produce collagen and other extracellular matrix components that form the scar tissue, providing structural integrity to the healing muscle. During this stage, fibrosis (scar tissue) closes the injured site and adheres the fascial layers together, causing fascial restrictions. I will discuss fascial restrictions in depth in the chapter on fascial restriction.
- **Angiogenesis**: New blood vessels form to provide necessary nutrients and oxygen to the regenerating tissue.

3. Maturation Stage: The Remodeling Phase

This final phase can last from several weeks to months and is focused on strengthening and refining the newly formed tissue:

- **Maturation of Muscle Fibers**: Newly formed muscle fibers mature and increase in size and strength.
- **Collagen Remodeling**: The initially disorganized collagen fibers become more organized and aligned along the lines of stress, which improves the tensile strength of the muscle.
- **Functional Recovery**: Gradually, the muscle regains its strength and functionality, although the healed muscle may never completely return to its pre-injury state.

Factors Influencing Muscle Healing

Several factors can affect the efficiency and outcome of muscle healing, including:

- **Age**: Younger individuals tend to heal faster than older adults.
- **Malnutrition**
- **Vitamins, Minerals, and Hormonal Imbalances**
- **Blood Supply**: Muscles with good blood supply generally heal better than those with less vascularization.
- **Re-injury**: Avoiding re-injury during the healing process is crucial for successful recovery.
- **Poor Posture and Body Mechanics**

Chronic Condition Vicious Cycle

According to the U.S. National Center for Health Statistics, a chronic condition is typically defined as one that persists for three months or more. In a chronic condition, the injured body part becomes trapped in a vicious cycle, continuously oscillating between the inflammation and proliferation stages. This cycle leads to excessive inflammation and fibrosis, which in turn cause muscle spasms and severe fascial restrictions. Deficiencies in vitamins and minerals can cause the body to remain stuck in the inflammation-proliferation cycle, preventing progression to the maturation stage. Additionally, excessive fibrosis and severe fascial restrictions can further complicate the issue, making it harder to break the cycle of chronic conditions.

Chronic Conditions

Inflammation

Increased Temperature
Loss of Function
Redness
Swelling
Pain

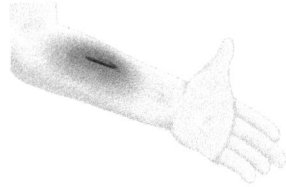

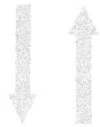

Proliferation

Fibrosis (Scar Tissue)
Fascia Restriction
Muscle Spasm
Trigger Points

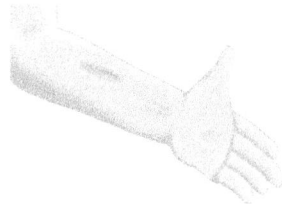

ASTR

This is the main reason for the failure of the biomedical model in treating chronic pain: it focuses on signs and symptoms instead of addressing fibrotic tissue, fascial restrictions, and imbalances in vitamins, minerals, and hormones.

Posture And Body Mechanics

Posture and body mechanics are important aspects that need to be addressed while treating musculoskeletal pain. Poor posture and poor body mechanics due to slouching or leaning forward for prolonged periods of time while using a computer, phone, or watching TV are risk factors and contributors to neck, back, shoulder, muscle, and joint pain. Poor posture is like having your car out of alignment; it leads to more wear and tear on one side of the tires compared to the other. Poor posture and body mechanics cause the same effect on your body, resulting in degeneration, strain, and sprain on the stressed parts.

Back Pain:

Slouching or leaning forward for prolonged periods of time (often due to sedentary lifestyles and desk jobs) can lead to back pain. This occurs due to placing uneven pressure and stress on the spine, leading to misalignment and strain on the spinal discs, muscles, and ligaments. Over time, this can cause or exacerbate conditions like herniated discs, sciatica, and chronic lower back pain.

Neck Pain

Forward head posture, such as looking down at a phone or computer screen, can strain the cervical vertebrae along with the supporting muscles and ligaments. This strain increases the risk of stiffness, soreness, and chronic neck pain.

Shoulder Pain

Forward shoulder posture can lead to pain, increased shoulder stiffness, decreased range of motion, and reduced mobility. Slumping or rounding shoulders not only stresses the shoulder joints but also the muscles and tendons. Over time, this can contribute to issues such as rotator cuff injuries, impingement, or even chronic conditions like bursitis and tendinitis.

Muscular Imbalances and Strain

Improper body mechanics, such as poor lifting techniques that utilize the back rather than the legs, can lead to muscle strain and sprains. Additionally, poor posture can cause certain muscles to work much harder than they should, leading to overuse and muscle fatigue. This imbalance can further contribute to pain and dysfunction.

Breathing and Circulation

Poor posture can also impact breathing and circulation. A slumped and slouching position compresses the chest and abdominal organs, potentially making breathing less efficient and slowing circulation. This decreases the ability to take full breaths, which can affect overall health and decrease energy levels due to reduced oxygen consumption.

The following are correct postures for walking, standing, sitting, using a computer, reading, and sleeping:

Posture and Body Mechanics Training Videos Available Online.

Standing Posture
1. **Visualize a string**: Imagine a string coming out of the top of your head, pulling you upward towards the ceiling.
2. **Core engagement**: Keep your belly button sucked in.
3. **Feet positioning**: Feet should be shoulder-width apart, with weight distributed through your heels.

Sitting Posture
1. **Visualize a string**: Imagine a string coming out of the top of your head, pulling you upward towards the ceiling.
2. **Engage your core**: Keep your belly button sucked in.

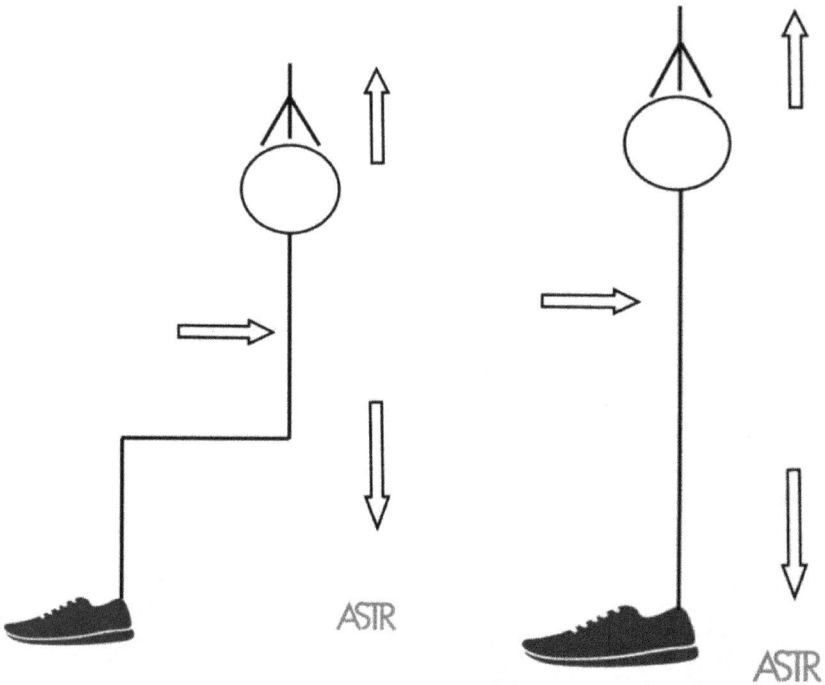

3. **Proper weight distribution**: Distribute your weight through your buttocks; keep your feet flat and shoulder-width apart.

Walking Posture

1. **Visualize a string**: Imagine a string coming out of the top of your head, pulling you upward towards the ceiling.
2. **Engage your core**: Suck your belly button in to stabilize your spine.
3. **Heel first**: Ensure your heel touches the ground first, then roll through to your toes.

General Tips

- **Start gradually**: Begin with short intervals, and progressively increase the duration you maintain these postures.
- **Be mindful**: Regularly check in with your body to ensure you're maintaining proper posture.

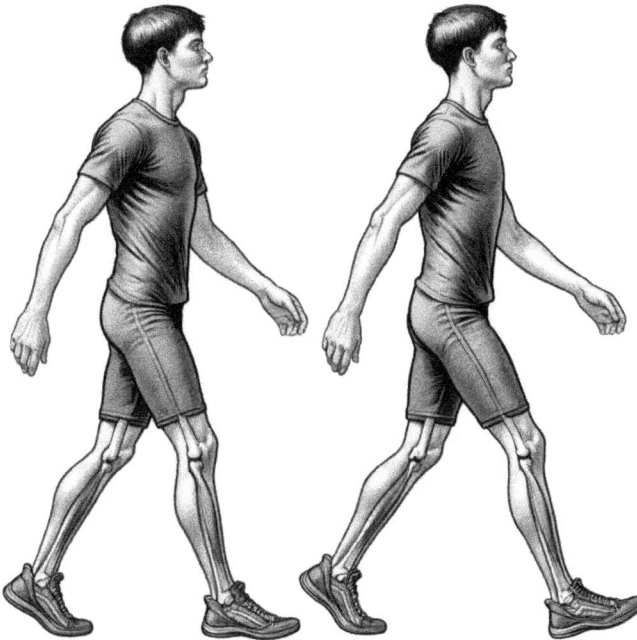

- **Create reminders**: Setting reminders can help you remember to adjust your posture throughout the day.

Correct Computer Posture

1. **Head and Neck Alignment**: Imagine a string pulling upward from the top of your head, keeping it level or slightly forward-facing and aligned with your torso. The neck should remain neutral, avoiding any tilting or twisting.

2. **Shoulder and Arm Position**: Shoulders should be relaxed, with upper arms hanging naturally at your sides. Elbows should be close to the body and bent at a 90-degree angle. Hands, wrists, and forearms should be straight, in-line, and roughly parallel to the floor, with forearms comfortably supported by armrests.

3. **Back Support**: Ensure your back is fully supported by the chair. Whether sitting upright or leaning back slightly, avoid twisting the back.

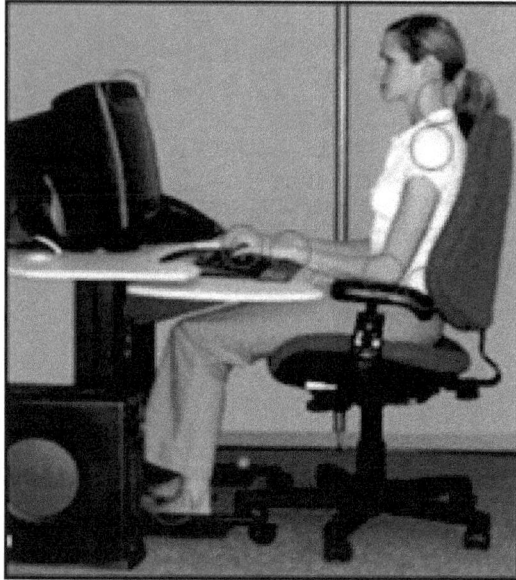

Image source: https://www.osha.gov/etools/computer-workstations

4. **Seat Positioning**: Thighs and hips should be supported by a well-padded seat, generally parallel to the floor. Knees should be at about the same height as the hips, with feet slightly forward.

5. **Foot Support**: Feet should rest fully on the floor. If the desk height is not adjustable and your feet do not comfortably reach the floor, use a footrest or a book to provide support.

6. **Monitor Setup**: Place the computer monitor directly in front of you, at eye level, to avoid straining your neck. The screen should be about an arm's length away, ensuring you do not have to tilt your head up, down, or sideways.

Additional Tips:

- **Adjust your chair**: Make sure your chair height and backrest are adjustable to fit your body dimensions.
- **Take breaks**: Regularly stand up, stretch, and walk around to relieve muscle tension and improve circulation.

- **Monitor brightness and distance**: Adjust the brightness of your monitor to a comfortable level to reduce eye strain. Ensure the monitor is neither too close nor too far for comfortable viewing.
- **Workspace layout**: Keep frequently used objects within easy reach to minimize reaching and twisting.

Implementing these practices can help reduce the risk of strain and discomfort. This contributes to a healthier, more productive work environment.

TV/Reading Posture

1. **Head and Neck Alignment**: Keep your head level or bent slightly forward, ensuring it remains in line with your torso. Your neck should be in a neutral position, not tilted to the side or excessively up or down.
2. **Eye Level**: Position your book or TV screen straight in front of you at eye level. This setup helps prevent neck strain by eliminating the need to look too far up, down, or to the side.
3. **Use a Reading Stand**: For reading, use a stand to hold your book. This reduces the strain on your arms and helps maintain a better neck posture.
4. **Shoulder Positioning**: Shoulders should be relaxed with upper arms hanging naturally at the sides. Avoid hunching or elevating your shoulders, which can lead to tension.
5. **Back Support**: Ensure your back is fully supported by the chair or sofa. Whether sitting upright or leaning back slightly, avoid twisting the back. This supports the natural curve of your spine and reduces lower back strain.
6. **Arm and Hand Relaxation:**Use a reading stand or rest your forearm on a pillow so that your hands and arms can rest comfortably. This reduces the strain of holding up a book for long periods.

Additional Recommendations:

- **Lighting**: Ensure adequate lighting for reading to avoid eye strain. The light source should come from behind you, ideally over your shoulder, to illuminate the page or screen without causing glare.

- **Seating Choice**: Choose a comfortable chair or sofa that supports your posture with cushions if necessary. Consider a recliner or a chair with an adjustable back for added comfort.
- **Take Breaks**: Regularly change your position and take breaks to stretch and move around. This helps reduce muscle fatigue and stiffness from prolonged sitting.

Implementing these recommendations can greatly enhance your viewing and reading experience, promoting better posture and reducing the risk of discomfort or injury.

Correct Back Sleeping Posture

1. **Avoid Stomach Sleeping**: Sleeping on your stomach can put excessive strain on your neck and back. Instead, opt for back sleeping as it

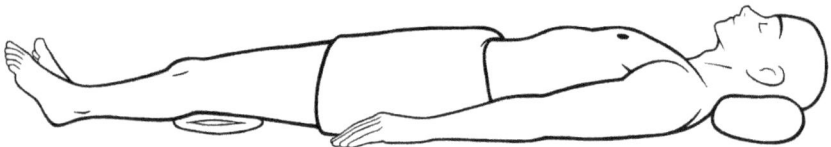

supports natural spinal alignment.

2. **Head and Neck Alignment**: Keep your head in a neutral position, avoiding any flexion (tilting forward) or excessive side bending. Use a semi-firm contoured memory foam pillow that supports the natural curve of your neck.

3. **Knee Support**: To maintain better spinal alignment and relieve pressure on your lower back, place a pillow under your knees. This helps flatten the lumbar region against the mattress and reduces stress on the spine.

Additional Tips:

- **Mattress Selection**: Choose a mattress that supports the contour of your spine. It should be firm enough to support your body but soft enough to allow for slight sinking of the heavier parts of your body.

- **Pillow Adjustments**: Ensure your pillow is not too high. It should just fill the space between your neck and the mattress to maintain proper alignment without lifting your head too high.
- **Relaxation Before Bed**: Engaging in relaxation techniques such as deep breathing before bed can help reduce muscle tension and promote better sleep.
- **Regular Review**: Evaluate your sleeping environment regularly to ensure it continues to meet your needs. This is especially important if you experience changes in health or comfort.

Implementing these practices not only improves your posture during sleep but can also enhance sleep quality. This helps prevent common discomforts associated with poor sleeping positions.

Correct Side Sleeping Posture

1. **Avoid Stomach Sleeping**: Sleeping on your stomach is discouraged due to potential neck and back strain. Side sleeping is a healthier alternative that supports better spinal alignment.
2. **Head and Neck Support**: Keep your head in a neutral position, avoiding any forward flexion or side bending. Use a semi-firm contoured memory foam pillow that adequately supports the natural curve of your neck. This aligns it with the rest of your spine.
3. **Knee and Hip Alignment**: Place a pillow thick enough between your knees to ensure that your hips, knees, and ankles are aligned. This prevents the upper leg from pulling the spine out of alignment and

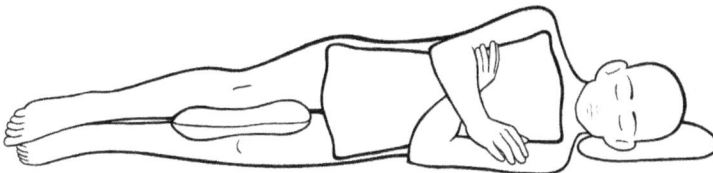

reduces stress on the hips and lower back.
4. **Avoid Trunk Twisting**: Maintain your trunk in a straight alignment with your hips and shoulders stacked directly above each other. This prevents

any twisting. Ensure your hips, knees, and ankles remain directly on top of each other.

5. **Use a Body Pillow**: A body pillow can be beneficial for side sleepers. It provides support for the arms and the entire body, helping to stabilize the trunk and prevent it from twisting during the night.

Additional Tips:

- **Pillow Adjustments**: Adjust the height and firmness of your pillow to ensure it fills the gap between your shoulder and the mattress. This helps maintain a straight neck and spine.
- **Mattress Firmness**: Choose a mattress that supports your body's weight while cushioning pressure points like hips and shoulders.
- **Regular Position Changes**: If feasible, alternate sides throughout the night to avoid overuse and strain on one side of your body.
- **Relaxation Techniques**: Engage in relaxing activities such as reading before bed to prepare your body for restful sleep.

Implementing these posture guidelines can greatly improve your sleep quality and contribute to overall spinal health.

Inflammatory Foods

Inflammatory foods are those that can contribute to or exacerbate inflammation in the body. Chronic inflammation is associated with a range of health issues, including heart disease, diabetes, joint pain, arthritis, and other chronic conditions. Identifying and reducing the intake of foods that promote inflammation can be beneficial for overall health. Here's a list of common inflammatory foods:

1. Sugar and High-Fructose Corn Syrup

High intakes of sugar and high-fructose corn syrup can exacerbate inflammation, oxidative stress, and insulin resistance. These sweeteners are prevalent in many processed foods and beverages. Such high consumption can increase inflammation and contribute to insulin resistance, thereby intensifying pain and swelling in joints. Common sources include soft drinks, candies, and various desserts.

Research by Sanchez et al. on the impact of carbohydrates, including glucose, on the phagocytic capacity of neutrophils in normal human subjects revealed that simple carbohydrates significantly decrease the capacity of neutrophils to engulf bacteria, with effects lasting for at least five hours post-ingestion. Engulfing bacteria is a process known as phagocytosis, where certain cells of the immune system, primarily phagocytes such as neutrophils and macrophages, ingest and destroy bacteria and other foreign particles. This suggests that glucose can induce internal inflammation lasting for five hours. Consuming three meals a day that contain refined carbs or simple sugars could subject the body to 15 hours of internal inflammation daily. Over a year, this means the body could be in a state of inflammation most of the time.

2. Artificial Trans Fats

These are considered the most unhealthy fats, created by adding hydrogen to unsaturated fats, which are found in margarine, spreads, and various processed foods. Trans fats are linked to increased inflammation, heart disease, and other health problems.

3. Vegetable and Seed Oils

Some vegetable oils that are high in omega-6 fatty acids and low in omega-3 fatty acids can contribute to inflammation if consumed in large quantities. Examples include corn, safflower, sunflower, and soybean oils. These oils tend to promote inflammation when consumed in large amounts, especially if the balance between omega-6 and omega-3 fatty acids in the diet is skewed towards omega-6s.

4. Refined Carbohydrates

Foods made from refined grains—like white bread, pasta, pastries, and many snacks—are stripped of their fiber and most nutrients during processing. When consumed, they can lead to rapid spikes in blood sugar and insulin levels.These spikes can, in turn, trigger an inflammatory response. Chronic high blood sugar levels can lead to insulin resistance, which is linked to further inflammation. Over time, this ongoing low-grade inflammation can contribute to the development of chronic diseases such as type 2 diabetes, heart disease, and other inflammatory conditions.

High intake of refined and simple carbohydrates has been associated with an increased risk of metabolic diseases and negative effects on mental health, including mood disorders like anxiety and depression. Reducing the intake of refined carbohydrates and replacing them with whole grain options can help manage and reduce inflammation.

5. Alcohol

Alcohol intake can have multiple negative effects on the body:

1. **Liver Damage**: Alcohol is metabolized by the liver. Excessive drinking can lead to conditions such as fatty liver, alcoholic hepatitis, fibrosis, and cirrhosis.
2. **Disruption of Bodily Processes**: Alcohol can interfere with the brain's communication pathways and affect the way the brain looks and works.

It also disrupts other bodily systems like the digestive system and immune system.

3. **Increased Risk of Cancer**: Drinking too much alcohol has been linked to an increased risk of several types of cancer, including liver, breast, throat, esophagus, and mouth cancer.

4. **Chronic Inflammation**: Alcohol can cause an inflammatory response in the body. Chronic alcohol use can lead to persistent inflammation, which can contribute to a variety of diseases.

6. Processed Meats

Processed meats, such as sausages, bacon, deli meats, and hot dogs, are known to contribute to inflammation due to several factors:

1. **High levels of saturated fats**: These can increase inflammation in the body, particularly when consumed in excess.

2. **Advanced glycation end products (AGEs)**: These compounds are formed when meats are cooked at high temperatures and can drive inflammation.

3. **Preservatives**: Many processed meats contain preservatives like sodium nitrate or nitrite, which have been linked to increased oxidative stress and inflammation in the body.

4. **High salt content**: Processed meats generally contain high amounts of salt, which can contribute to increased blood pressure and inflammation.

The regular consumption of processed meats has been associated with an increased risk of chronic diseases such as heart disease, type 2 diabetes, and certain types of cancer, all of which are linked to chronic inflammation. Reducing the intake of processed meats can be beneficial for reducing overall inflammation and improving health.

Case Study 3: **Knee Pain and Blood Sugar Decreased from 500 to 89**

Diagnosis: Diabetes and knee pain
Symptoms: Constant 8/10 aching knee pain, very stiff limping gait, fatigue,

inability to sleep more than 3 hours at night, knee swelling, difficulty with walking and stair climbing, anxiety and depression, and walking with a cane.

Previous Failed Treatments: Partial knee replacement, total knee replacement, knee arthroscopy, knee manipulation surgery, physical therapy, cortisone shots, massage therapy, pain medication, and diabetic medication.

Length of Injury: 4 years

Pain Level on a Scale of 0 to 10: 8-10/10

Treatment: Treatment included releasing fibrotic tissue, addressing fascia restrictions, decreasing inflammation, improving ergonomics, implementing an anti-inflammatory diet, and addressing vitamin, mineral, and hormonal imbalances.

Outcome: Symptoms resolved

Case Study 4: Knee Swelling and Alcohol Consumption

I treated an Italian patient who suffered from chronic knee pain accompanied by severe swelling. During her treatment, she responded well when I released fascial restrictions and fibrotic tissue in her knee (I will explain the fascial restrictions and fibrotic tissues in the following chapters). However, her pain relief typically lasted only a day after each treatment. During an evaluation of her diet, she mentioned that she drinks a glass of alcohol every night. I suggested that her severe knee swelling could be due to her alcohol consumption. Initially, the patient was reluctant to stop drinking, so I persuaded her to abstain from alcohol for just three days and to monitor her knee swelling. At the follow-up visits, I observed that her knee inflammation had subsided, and she reported that she had not consumed alcohol since our last treatment.

Case Study 5: Trigger Fingers and Refined Carbohydrates

I treated a Filipino patient who had suffered from trigger fingers for over three years. After releasing the fibrotic tissue and fascial restrictions in his fingers, he was able to make a fist without his fingers locking. The patient was doing great for a week, but then he returned, indicating that his fingers had started to lock again. I performed a nutritional analysis and noticed that he consumed refined carbohydrates and fried food almost daily. I prescribed an anti-inflammatory diet and advised him to stop eating refined carbs and fried foods. During his follow-up visits, the patient reported that his treatment relief lasted as long as he avoided refined carbohydrates and fried foods.

Anti-Inflammatory Diet

Switching from a diet high in inflammatory foods to one that includes more anti-inflammatory options can have profound health benefits. Here are some anti-inflammatory food choices:

- **Fruits and Vegetables**: Loaded with antioxidants, fruits and vegetables can reduce inflammation. Berries, oranges, and leafy greens are particularly beneficial.
- **Omega-3 Fatty Acids**: Found in fatty fish like salmon, mackerel, and sardines, as well as in flaxseeds and walnuts. Omega-3 fats are known for their anti-inflammatory effects.
- **Whole Grains**: Whole grains contain more fiber, which has been shown to reduce levels of C-reactive protein, a marker of inflammation in the blood.
- **Nuts**: Almonds, walnuts, and other nuts are great sources of inflammation-fighting healthy fats.
- **Spices and Herbs**: Many spices and herbs like turmeric, ginger, and garlic have potent anti-inflammatory properties.

I developed the ASTR Diet as the result of 15 years of dedicated research and personal experience, driven by a mission to help individuals overcome chronic inflammation and achieve lasting health. This anti-inflammatory approach focuses on eliminating processed foods, toxins, and harmful ingredients while embracing nutrient-dense, wholesome foods that support the body's natural healing processes. The ASTR Diet is more than a dietary plan, it is a lifestyle designed to restore balance and vitality. For a comprehensive guide to this transformative approach, including practical tips, meal plans, and recipes, I invite you to explore my book, **Eat to Heal**. Here is the QR code for the book:

EAT TO HEAL

The ASTR Diet: Unlock the Healing Power of Food to End Sickness and Thrive

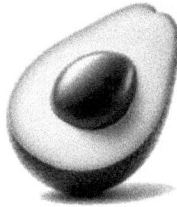

- Achieve Lasting Weight Loss
- Reverse Chronic Diseases Naturally
- Heal Inflammation and Pain
- Boost Energy and Vitality
- 3 Steps to Transform Your Health

Dr. Joseph Jacobs, DPT, ACN

Stress Management

Research studies showing that stress has consistently demonstrated its impact on various biological systems, potentially leading to a range of health issues. Here's a summary of how stress affects different parts of the body based on scientific studies:

1. Cardiovascular Effects: Stress may increase heart rate, blood pressure, and oxygen demand on the heart. It can also lead to vasoconstriction, increased blood lipids, and blood clotting issues, contributing to atherosclerosis and increased risk of heart attack and stroke.
2. Metabolic Effects: Stress can cause the liver to produce extra blood sugar (glucose), increasing the risk of developing type 2 diabetes
3. Gastrointestinal Effects: Stress can disrupt normal digestive function, leading to issues like heartburn, acid reflux, diarrhea, constipation, and stomach pain
4. Musculoskeletal Effects: Stress can cause muscles to tense up, leading to headaches, back pain, shoulder pain, and body aches.
5. Reproductive Effects: In men, stress can lower testosterone levels and interfere with sperm production and sexual function. In women, stress can disrupt the menstrual cycle.
6. Immune System Effects: Chronic stress can weaken the immune system, increasing susceptibility to infections.
7. Neurological/Psychological Effects: Stress can contribute to conditions like anxiety, depression, and insomnia. It can also impair cognitive function like memory and concentration

Stress and muscle tension are closely related, and understanding this relationship can help in managing both effectively. Here's how stress leads to muscle tension and the potential long-term effects if it remains unaddressed:

\

Mechanisms of Muscle Tension Due to Stress

1. **Fight-or-Flight Response:** When you experience stress, your body's fight-or-flight response is triggered. This response prepares your body to either fight or flee from perceived threats. As part of this response, your muscles tense up, readying you for physical action. This was useful in ancient times when physical threats were common. However, in

modern life, this response can be triggered by non-physical stresses like deadlines, traffic, or personal conflicts.

2. **Cortisol Release**: Stress stimulates the release of cortisol, a hormone that increases glucose in the bloodstream and enhances the brain's use of glucose. Cortisol also restricts functions that are non-essential in a fight-or-flight situation, such as the immune response. High cortisol levels can lead to sustained muscle tension.

3. **Neuromuscular Reaction**: Stress affects the nervous system, which controls muscle activation. Under stress, the nervous system may keep muscles in a partly contracted state for prolonged periods.

Effects of Chronic Muscle Tension

1. **Pain and Discomfort**: Prolonged muscle tension can lead to muscle pain and discomfort, which might manifest as back pain, headaches, or neck pain. Tension-type headaches, one of the most common types of headaches, are directly linked to muscle tension in the neck and scalp.

2. **Reduced Mobility**: Over time, chronic muscle tension can reduce joint mobility. This stiffness can affect your posture and the way you move, potentially leading to mechanical imbalances and injury.

3. **Fibrotic tissue & Trigger Points**: Chronic tension can lead to the development of fibrotic tissue and trigger points—small knots that form in muscles and may cause pain in other parts of the body. These are often tender to the touch and can contribute to pain patterns seen in conditions like myofascial pain syndrome.

4. **Fatigue**: Muscles that are constantly under stress consume energy even when you're at rest. This can lead to muscle fatigue, which reduces your energy levels overall and can impact your physical performance.

Effective Strategies for Managing Stress

Managing stress effectively is crucial for maintaining both physical and mental health. Here are some practical tips for managing stress:

1. **Identify Stressors**: Keep a journal to identify the situations that create the most stress and how you respond to them. Noting patterns can help you find better coping strategies.
2. **Regular Physical Activity**: Exercise can help alleviate stress by producing endorphins (chemicals in the brain that act as natural painkillers) and improving your ability to sleep, which can reduce stress.
3. **Mindfulness and Meditation**: Techniques such as meditation, deep breathing exercises, and mindfulness can help melt away stress. Start with just a few minutes a day and increase the duration as you feel more comfortable.
4. **Time Management**: Improve your time management skills to avoid feeling overwhelmed. Prioritize tasks, set boundaries, and break projects into manageable steps.
5. **Establish Boundaries**: In today's digital world, it's important to know when to turn off electronic devices. Set boundaries for work and social interactions to ensure personal time for relaxation.
6. **Nourish Your Body**: Eat a healthy diet. Well-nourished bodies are better prepared to cope with stress, so be mindful of what you eat.
7. **Sleep Adequately**: Ensure you get enough sleep. Lack of sleep is a significant contributor to stress. Most adults need 7-9 hours per night.
8. **Connect with Others**: Share your stress and concerns with friends or family members. Social connections can help you feel understood and supported.
9. **Practice Relaxation Techniques**: Engage in activities you enjoy, such as reading, yoga, or listening to music. Try relaxation techniques like progressive muscle relaxation or visualization.
10. **Seek Professional Help**: If your stress levels become too overwhelming, consider seeking professional help. Biopsychosocial therapist can help you learn how to manage stress effectively.

By incorporating these stress management tips into your life, you can find ways to reduce your stress levels and improve your overall well-being.

Meditation

Focused Breathing (Eyes Open or Closed)
- **Procedure**: Take a slow, deep breath in and out through your nose, filling your lungs with air.
- **Focus**: Concentrate on your breathing. If your mind wanders, gently redirect it to focus on your breathing.
- **Purpose**: This meditation breathing exercise can be used to help you go to sleep.
- **Session Duration**: 1 to 10 minutes, or as needed throughout the day.

Breathing Exercise I (Eyes Open)
- **Setting**: Can be done anywhere.
- **Procedure**:
  1. Take a slow, deep breath through your nose, filling your lungs with air.
  2. Hold your breath for 5 to 15 seconds.
  3. Exhale slowly through your nose.
  4. Repeat this process 20 times per session.
- **Focus**: Concentrate on your breathing and redirect your focus if your mind wanders.
- **Frequency**: Perform 4-5 sessions per day.

Breathing Exercise II (Eyes Closed)
- **Setting**: Perform this exercise in a quiet room.
- **Position**: Sit in a comfortable chair with back support, rest your arms on a pillow in your lap, and keep your feet flat on the floor (shoulder width apart).
- **Procedure**:
  1. Take a slow, deep breath in through your nose.
  2. Hold your breath for 5 to 15 seconds.
  3. Exhale slowly through your nose.
  4. Repeat this process 20 times per session.
- **Focus**: Concentrate on your breathing and redirect your focus if your mind wanders.

- **Frequency**: Perform 4-5 sessions per day.

Breathing Exercise III (Eyes Closed)
- **Setting**: Perform this exercise in a quiet room.
- **Position**: Sit in a comfortable chair with back support, rest your arms on a pillow in your lap, and keep your feet flat on the floor (shoulder width apart).
- **Procedure**:
  1. Take a slow, deep breath in through your nose.
  2. Hold your breath for 5 to 15 seconds.
  3. Exhale slowly through your mouth while making a vibration sound.
  4. Repeat this process 40 times per session.
- **Focus**: Concentrate on your breathing and redirect your focus if your mind wanders.
- **Frequency**: Perform 2-3 sessions per day.

Conclusion

Stress plays a significant role in chronic pain, often amplifying its intensity and duration. Long-term stress leads to physiological changes that heighten pain sensitivity, disrupt healing, and increase inflammation. While the strategies outlined in this chapter offer practical guidance for managing general stress, emotional challenges such as chronic anxiety, depression, and post-traumatic stress disorder (PTSD) require more specialized attention than can be fully covered here.

For readers struggling with ongoing emotional distress or trauma-related issues, I highly recommend exploring my companion book *Beating Anxiety and Depression: 14 Natural Secrets to a Happier Life*. This comprehensive guide is designed specifically to address deeper emotional conditions by providing clear, evidence-based approaches that target the biological, psychological, and lifestyle factors driving anxiety, depression, and PTSD.

Due to the complexity and depth of mental health topics, it is impossible to adequately cover chronic anxiety, depression, or PTSD in just one chapter.

Beating Anxiety and Depression serves as a dedicated resource, offering practical tools and insights to empower readers on their journey toward lasting emotional wellness. If chronic stress, anxiety, depression, or unresolved trauma contributes to your experience of pain, this book will serve as an essential step toward holistic healing and well-being.

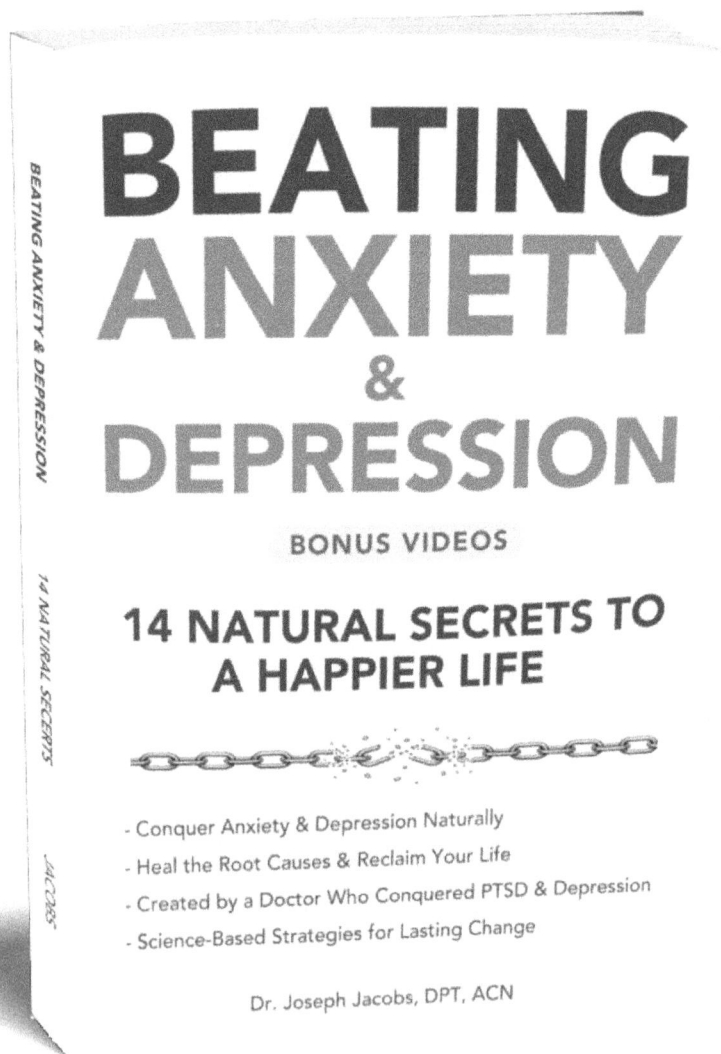

BEATING ANXIETY & DEPRESSION

BONUS VIDEOS

14 NATURAL SECRETS TO A HAPPIER LIFE

- Conquer Anxiety & Depression Naturally
- Heal the Root Causes & Reclaim Your Life
- Created by a Doctor Who Conquered PTSD & Depression
- Science-Based Strategies for Lasting Change

Dr. Joseph Jacobs, DPT, ACN

Fibrotic Tissue

Do you tend to slouch or hunch forward when using your phone or computer? Believe it or not, poor posture can cause fibrotic tissue (scar tissue) to build up in the neck and shoulders. If possible, place your hand on the back of your shoulder, close to your neck, and press firmly. If you notice a hard knot, it's possible that you have fibrotic tissue (scar tissue) as a result of poor posture. Since we cannot visually see internal fibrotic tissue, it is often overlooked and ignored. Our muscles should act like a rubber band, contracting and relaxing to encourage a full range of motion in the joint. However, fibrotic tissue acts like a knot in the rubber band, limiting its full range of motion. Patients with fibrotic tissue may experience pain and decreased range of motion. If left untreated, this condition can lead to nerve damage, chronic pain, and may even require surgery.

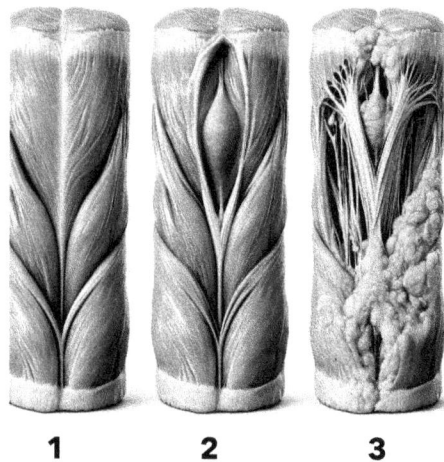

1   2   3

Image Explanation
1. **Healthy, intact muscle:** An illustration showing the muscle fibers in their natural, unbroken state.
2. **Muscle with tear:** An illustration depicting a clear gap in the tissue where the muscle fibers are disrupted and separated.
3. **Muscle with fibrotic tissue:** An illustration of a muscle with a tear and dense, scar-like fibrotic tissue contrasting with the normal muscle fibers.

Fibroblasts

Fibroblasts are a type of cell that are essential for wound healing and play a critical role in the maintenance and repair of connective tissues throughout the body. They are the most common cells of connective tissue in animals. They are typically active during the proliferation phase of the healing process. Fibroblasts are a type of cell most commonly found within connective tissues in animals. They play a crucial role in the structural framework of tissues by producing and maintaining the extracellular matrix, which is the complex scaffold of proteins and other substances that support cells. Fibroblasts are responsible for producing key components of this matrix, including collagen, fibronectin, and elastin, which help provide structural integrity and elasticity to tissues.

During wound healing or in response to injury, fibroblasts are activated and multiply. They are crucial in the healing process as they migrate to the site of injury, where they produce collagen and other extracellular matrix components to form fibrotic tissue and repair the damaged tissue. In pathological conditions, fibroblasts can become overly active. This leads to excessive deposition of connective and fibrotic tissue, which can disrupt normal tissue architecture and function.

Here are some key functions and characteristics of fibroblasts:

1. **Tissue Repair and Maintenance**: Fibroblasts produce and secrete collagen and other extracellular matrix proteins that form the structural framework for tissues such as skin, tendons, and ligaments.
2. **Wound Healing**: During the process of wound healing, fibroblasts are activated and migrate to the site of injury. They proliferate and produce collagen and other fibers, which help in closing and healing the wound.
3. **Fibrotic Tissue Formation**: In the proliferation stages of wound healing, fibroblasts help in the formation of fibrotic tissue by depositing excess collagen. This can sometimes lead to the overproduction of fibrosis.
4. **Role in Diseases**: Abnormal function and activation of fibroblasts can contribute to a variety of pathological conditions, including fibrosis

(excessive fibrous connective tissue formation) and autoimmune diseases such as rheumatoid arthritis and systemic sclerosis. Fibroblasts can also differentiate into myofibroblasts, especially during wound healing, which possess contractile capabilities similar to muscle cells, aiding in the contraction of the wound.

Fibrosis

Fibrosis is defined by the overgrowth, hardening, and/or scarring of various tissues and is attributed to the excess deposition of extracellular matrix components, including collagen. Fibrosis characterizes a pathological state of excessive tissue repair where there is an overgrowth, hardening, and scarring of tissue primarily due to the excessive deposition of extracellular matrix components such as collagen. This process can affect virtually any tissue in the body, leading to significant organ dysfunction depending on the site and severity of the fibrotic response.

Fibrosis often results from chronic inflammatory reactions triggered by a variety of stimuli. These can include:

- **Poor posture and body mechanics:** This is considered a repetitive strain injury due to prolonged poor posture and body mechanics, which cause muscle strain and tendon sprains. This strain leads to inflammation, and eventually, the body builds excessive fibrotic tissue.
- **Persistent infections:** Where ongoing microbial presence provokes a sustained immune response.
- **Autoimmune reactions:** Where the body's immune system mistakenly attacks its own tissues.
- **Allergic responses:** Which can cause chronic inflammation due to repeated exposure to allergens.
- **Chemical insults:** Such as exposure to toxins or irritants that cause tissue damage and subsequent fibrotic repair.
- **Radiation:** Which can damage cells and extracellular matrix, leading to scarring and fibrosis.

- **Physical tissue injury:** From events like trauma or surgery, which initiates the healing process that can sometimes lead to excessive scar tissue formation if the healing process is dysregulated.

The fibrotic process involves complex signaling pathways and cellular interactions, primarily involving fibroblasts, as mentioned earlier. These fibroblasts play a key role in synthesizing and remodeling the extracellular matrix during both normal tissue repair and pathological fibrosis.

Understanding the function of fibroblasts and regulating their activity can be crucial for managing and treating various conditions involving tissue repair and fibrosis. Fibrotic tissue, often known as scar tissue, is a type of connective tissue that forms during the wound healing process, particularly during the proliferation stage. It mainly consists of collagen, a protein that provides structural strength. While essential for repairing damaged areas, excessive fibrotic tissue can lead to muscle or joint pain and restricted range of motion.

Characteristics of Fibrotic Tissue

1. **Composition**: Fibrotic tissue has a higher density of collagen fibers compared to normal tissue. These fibers are often more disorganized and aligned differently than in the original tissue, which can affect the flexibility and functionality of the area.
2. **Elasticity**: Scar tissue is less elastic and more fibrous than the original tissue. This can lead to stiffness and restricted movement, especially if the fibrosis occurs near joints.
3. **Vascularity**: Fibrotic tissue typically has fewer blood vessels than the original tissue, making it appear paler and potentially leading to a slower metabolic rate in that area.
4. **Sensory Nerves**: fibrotic tissue may have fewer sensory nerves, which can result in areas of numbness or altered sensation.

Causes of Fibrosis

Fibrosis can result from a variety of conditions and scenarios, including:

- **Injury:** Following trauma or surgery, fibrotic tissue develops as part of the natural healing process to close the wound site. If the wound site remains open, it is susceptible to infection. Fibrotic tissues are crucial for our survival. However, the problem arises when excessive fibrotic tissue forms, which can compress blood vessels and nerves, limit range of motion, and cause pain.
- **Chronic Inflammation**: Diseases that cause long-term inflammation can lead to excessive fibrotic tissue formation. This is seen in conditions such as rheumatoid arthritis, osteoarthritis, fibromyalgia, ankylosing spondylitis, psoriatic arthritis, systemic lupus erythematosus, tendonitis, bursitis, and various autoimmune diseases.
- **Repeated Injury or Irritation**: Areas of the body that undergo repeated stress or injury can become chronically inflamed and subsequently fibrotic.
- **Disease Processes**: Certain diseases can promote fibrosis. These include conditions such as liver cirrhosis from chronic hepatitis or liver damage, pulmonary fibrosis in the lungs, and systemic diseases like scleroderma, which affects connective tissue.
- **Stretching:** Frequent and intense stretching can lead to inflammation and overstimulation of fibroblasts. This can result in increased collagen production and potentially lead to excessive fibrotic tissue formation within the tendons.
- **Poor posture and body mechanics:** This is considered a repetitive strain injury due to prolonged poor posture and body mechanics, which cause muscle strain and tendon sprains. This strain leads to inflammation, and eventually, the body builds excessive fibrotic tissue.

Impact of Fibrotic Tissue

Excessive fibrotic tissue in the body can have a range of detrimental effects, impacting various organs and systems. Fibrosis is essentially the thickening and scarring of connective tissue, usually resulting from a healing process in response to injury or long-term inflammation. Here are some key impacts of excessive fibrotic tissue:

- **Nerve damage:** If excessive fibrotic tissue compresses nerve cells, it could cause numbness, tingling sensations, or permanent nerve damage, resulting in loss of function and sensation. This can occur in conditions such as sciatica, carpal tunnel syndrome, and others.
- **Chronic Pain:** Fibrosis can lead to chronic pain, especially when it affects muscles, joints, or tissues involved in movement. Conditions such as Dupuytren's contracture, back pain, neck pain, sciatica, carpal tunnel syndrome, bursitis, tendonitis, plantar fasciitis, frozen shoulder, tension headaches, and trigger finger are examples where fibrosis can significantly contribute to discomfort and mobility issues.
- **Mobility Issues**: In muscles, tendons, and ligaments, fibrosis can restrict movement, leading to stiffness and pain. Typically, our muscles behave like a rubber band, stretching and elongating as they contract and relax. However, when fibrotic tissue is present in the muscle, it acts like a knot that limits muscle contraction, reduces range of motion, and causes pain.
- **Reduced Functionality**: Fibrotic tissue is less flexible than normal tissue, which can lead to impaired function of the affected organ or area. For example, in the lungs (as in pulmonary fibrosis), this can lead to difficulty breathing and decreased oxygen intake.
- **Organ Dysfunction**: In organs like the liver (cirrhosis), heart (cardiac fibrosis), and kidneys (renal fibrosis), excessive fibrotic tissue can disrupt normal function. This can result in a significant decrease in the organ's ability to perform its essential tasks, such as filtering blood, pumping blood, or metabolizing substances.
- **Increased Risk of Complications**: Fibrotic changes can increase the risk of further complications. For instance, liver cirrhosis, which involves fibrosis or scarring of the liver, can lead to complications such as portal hypertension and visceral bleeding.
- **Impaired Healing and Regeneration**: Excessive fibrosis can interfere with the normal healing process, as scar tissue can replace normal, healthy tissue, leading to prolonged or incomplete recovery.
- **Restricted Movement**: In cases where fibrosis affects the skin, muscles, or connective tissues (such as in scleroderma or after severe burns), it can lead to reduced mobility due to stiff and tightened tissues.

- **Aesthetic Concerns**: On the skin, fibrotic tissue can cause cosmetic concerns, especially if the scarring is extensive or occurs in highly visible areas.

You can watch the following case studies and live recorded treatments using the barcode below:

<u>Case Study 6:</u> **20 Years of Fibromyalgia, Jaw Pain and Headaches**
Diagnosis: Fibromyalgia, jaw pain, and headaches
Symptoms: Jaw pain, daily headaches, chronic pain, fatigue and stiffness, low energy, body pain, and jaw clicking.
Previous Failed Treatments: Dentist and medical doctors
Length of Injury: 20 years
Pain Level on a Scale of 0 to 10:
Treatment: Treatment included releasing fibrotic tissue, addressing fascia restrictions, decreasing inflammation, improving ergonomics, implementing an anti-inflammatory diet, and addressing vitamin, mineral, and hormonal imbalances.
Outcome: Symptoms resolved

<u>Case Study 7:</u> **5 Months of Ankle Pain**
Diagnosis: Ankle pain
Symptoms: Constant ankle pain (2-3/10), increased pain with exercises
Previous Failed Treatments:
Length of Injury: 5 months
Pain Level on a Scale of 0 to 10: 2-8/10
Treatment: Treatment included releasing fibrotic tissue, addressing fascia restrictions, decreasing inflammation, improving ergonomics, implementing an anti-inflammatory diet, and addressing vitamin, mineral, and hormonal imbalances.
Outcome: Symptoms resolved

Case Study 8: 2+ Years of Bilateral Plantar Fasciitis
Diagnosis: Bilateral plantar fasciitis
Symptoms: Constant bilateral foot pain (5-8/10), increased pain with weight bearing, inability to walk, very stiff limping gait, sharp/throbbing/aching bilateral foot pain, Achilles pain, and pain that increases in the morning with the first few steps.
Previous Failed Treatments: Podiatrist, neurologist, rheumatologist, foot boot, foot cast, foot orthotics, and physical therapy.
Length of Injury: 2+ years
Pain Level on a Scale of 0 to 10: 8-10/10
Treatment: Treatment included releasing fibrotic tissue, addressing fascia restrictions, decreasing inflammation, improving ergonomics, implementing an anti-inflammatory diet, and addressing vitamin, mineral, and hormonal imbalances.
Outcome: Symptoms resolved

Ineffective Methods for Breaking Down Fibrotic Tissue

Fibrotic tissue, due to its thickness and hardness, requires firm mechanical force to break down. An understanding of the physiology of fibrosis shows that certain approaches are ineffective for breaking down fibrotic tissue. These include massage, foam rollers, manual therapy, Gua Sha, instrument-assisted soft tissue mobilization, stretching, and exercises.

1. **Foam rollers:** These approaches typically provide only superficial pressure on the tissue. In many cases, fibrotic tissue is located deep within muscles, such as in the hamstrings, quadriceps, and gluteus muscles, where it can be up to 2 inches deep. This renders foam rollers ineffective for reaching and treating these areas.
2. **Deep tissue massage:** Involves the therapist using their hands, knuckles, and/or elbows to reach deeper layers of muscle. However, due to the width and diameter of the therapist's knuckles and elbows, it is difficult to

penetrate deep tissues and provide consistent forces necessary to break down deep fibrotic tissue

3. **Manual therapy:** Similar to massage, manual therapy often involves using the knuckles, elbows, or hands to reach deeper tissues. However, the relatively large diameter of the therapist's hands and elbows may limit their ability to penetrate deeply enough to effect physiological changes in fibrotic tissues located deep within muscles.

4. **Exercises and Stretching:** Do not exert sufficient mechanical force on fibrotic tissue to break it down; they simply cause movement in the muscle.

5. **Myofascial release:** Involves applying gentle, sustained pressure to the superficial connective tissue, which may not exert enough mechanical force to break down scar tissue or reach deeply enough to affect deep fibrosis.

6. **Gua Sha and Instrument-Assisted Soft Tissue Mobilization:** These techniques involve tools that might resemble rods or a butter knife, used to apply horizontal superficial force on the skin. Like manual therapy, they fail

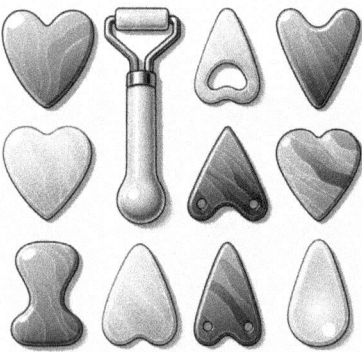

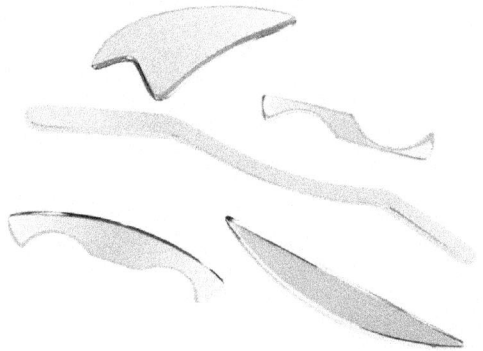

Instrument Assisted Soft Tissue Mobilization (IASTM)

Gua Sha

to penetrate deeply enough to alter fibrotic tissue effectively. This is like trying to unscrew a deep-set screw in a car with a screwdriver that is too short; it simply cannot reach deep enough to be effective.

The Solution

Analyzing and testing current approaches that claim to break down fibrotic tissue led me to realize that it is physiologically impossible to effectively target both superficial and deep fibrotic tissue with these methods. This realization was the turning point that inspired the invention of ergonomically designed ASTR instruments. These instruments are specifically created to address both superficial and deep fibrotic tissue, capable of penetrating up to 2 inches deep to break down adhesions.

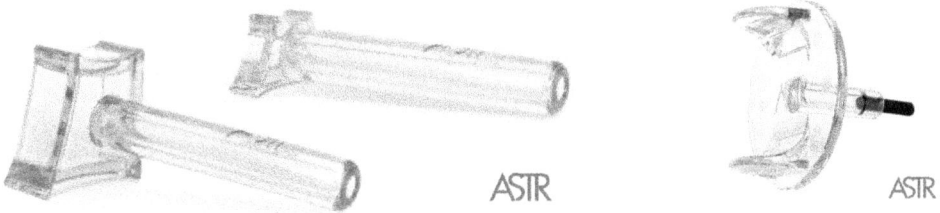

ASTR

ASTR

Summary

In cases of chronic conditions, the affected body part often remains caught in a relentless cycle, repeatedly fluctuating between inflammation and proliferation. This cycle results in significant inflammation and fibrosis, leading to muscle spasms and intense fascial restrictions. Nutritional deficiencies in vitamins and minerals may keep the body stuck in this cycle, blocking the progression to the maturation stage. Moreover, the presence of excessive fibrosis and intense fascial restrictions can further exacerbate the situation, making it more challenging to interrupt the ongoing cycle of chronic conditions.

This persistent issue underpins the biomedical model's inability to effectively treat chronic pain, as it primarily concentrates on symptoms rather than addressing underlying issues such as fibrotic tissue, fascial restrictions, and hormonal and nutritional imbalances.

Fascial Restrictions

The fascial system, an integral component of the body's connective tissue network, plays a crucial role in supporting and connecting all bodily structures. Here's a comprehensive overview of the fascial system:

What is Fascia?

Next time you buy meat, look for the white filaments in it; those are the fascia

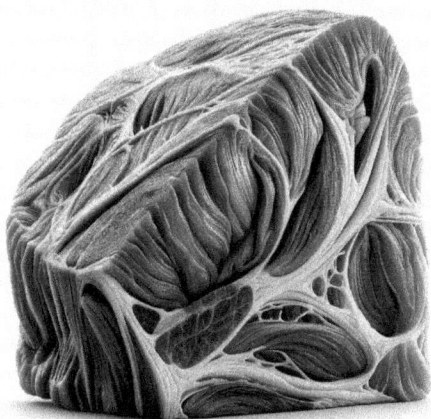

The white filaments in the meat are the fascia layers

layers. Fascia is a dense, tough tissue that extends throughout the body in a three-dimensional web from head to toe. It surrounds and interpenetrates every muscle, bone, nerve, blood vessel, and organ. Fascia is primarily made up of collagen fibers, which provide it with both flexibility and strength. Fascia is a complex network of connective tissue that extends throughout the body and plays a crucial role in supporting and protecting bodily structures.

Key Attributes of the Fascial System

The fascia system, a continuous network of connective tissue that envelops and interconnects every structure in the body, plays a critical role in maintaining overall health and physical integrity. Here are the key attributes of the fascial system:

1. Ubiquity and Continuity
Fascia is present throughout the entire body. It wraps around and interconnects muscles, bones, organs, nerves, and blood vessels, forming a seamless web that extends from head to toe. This continuity is crucial for the integration and coordination of bodily structures and functions.

2. Structural Support and Protection
Fascia provides a framework that supports the body's structures. It helps maintain the position of organs, enables the transmission of muscular force, and protects internal structures from physical trauma.

3. Flexibility and Elasticity
Despite its strength, fascia is also highly flexible and elastic. This allows it to stretch and move without restriction, accommodating movements of muscles and joints while returning to its original shape.

4. Sensory Role
Fascia is richly innervated with nerve endings, making it an important sensory organ. These nerves are responsible for proprioception (the sense of body position and movement) and the perception of pain. This sensory role is essential for maintaining posture and physical coordination.

5. Fluid Transport
The fascial network plays a role in the circulation of fluids throughout the body, including blood and lymphatic fluid. It facilitates the transport of nutrients and waste products to and from cells.

6. Metabolic Function
Fascia can store energy in the form of fat and water, and it also provides pathways for inflammation and healing. The extracellular matrix within the fascia contains cells that can respond to and influence metabolic processes.

7. Adaptability

Fascia is highly adaptable and responsive to physical and emotional stimuli. Chronic stress, injury, or poor postural habits can lead to changes in the fascial structures, sometimes leading to restrictions and pain.

8. Pathway for Force Transmission

Fascia transmits mechanical tension generated by muscle activity or external forces across the body. This distribution of force helps in reducing local stress on muscles and joints and enhances overall movement efficiency.

9. Compartmentalization

Through deeper layers, such as the deep fascia, it compartmentalizes sections of the body, segregating groups of muscles and other structures into functional units. This compartmentalization aids in organizing the body architecturally and facilitates effective movement and function.

These attributes illustrate why the fascial system is integral not only to movement and stability but also to the general health and well-being of the body. Understanding and addressing fascial health is crucial in sports, rehabilitation, and general physical maintenance.

Layers of the Fascial System

There are several distinct layers of fascia, each with its specific function and characteristics. Understanding these layers helps in appreciating the complexity of human anatomy and the integration of bodily functions. Here's a detailed explanation of the different fascia layers:

1. Superficial Fascia (Subcutaneous Tissue)

Location: The superficial fascia layer is like a Spider-Man suit covering the whole body. Just below the skin, above the deeper layers of fascia.This layer separates the skin from the musculoskeletal system, allowing for normal sliding between the muscles and skin.

Composition: Consists of loose connective tissue and fat. This layer varies in thickness across different parts of the body and from person to person. Many nerve fibers are observed, and in some regions, the superficial fascia splits, forming specialized compartments. The collagen fibers are arranged irregularly. It consists of different layers that can slide over one another. The superficial fascia layer consists of two to three layers on top of each other

Functions: Acts as a water storage medium, provides insulation and padding, and allows the skin to move freely over underlying structures. It also serves as a conduit for nerves and blood vessels as they pass to and from the skin.

2. Deep Fascia

Location: Surrounds and infuses with muscles, bones, nerves, and blood vessels to the level of the dermis.

Composition: Denser than superficial fascia, this layer is made of tightly packed collagen fibers running in a parallel arrangement. It forms a fibrous sheath that encloses muscles and divides them into groups. Each

Musclar Fascia Layers

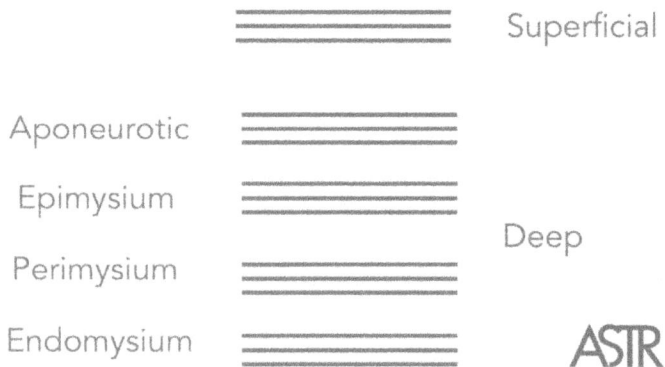

Superficial

Aponeurotic

Epimysium

Deep

Perimysium

Endomysium

ASTR

subdivision of the deep fascia layer consists of two to three layers on top of each other.

Functions: Provides an extensive area for muscle attachment, enhances force transmission across muscles, and maintains structural integrity. The deep fascia also separates different functional areas of muscles, allowing them to operate independently.

Division of Deep Fascia:

- **Aponeurotic Fascia:** Surrounds groups of muscles. It consists of 2 or 3 layers of unidirectional collagen fibers, with each layer separated by loose connective tissue. Composed of 80% collagen fibers and only 1% elastic fibers. This fascia helps keep a group of muscles in place or serves as the insertion point for a broad muscle.
- **Epimysial Fascia:** Surrounds the entire muscle. It is formed of type I and III collagen and is specific to each muscle. It contains approximately 15% elastic fibers. The epimysium is free to glide due to being separated from the aponeurotic fascia by an external layer of loose connective tissue. It is thinner than the aponeurotic fascia and is also separated from the perimysial fascia by an internal layer of loose connective tissue. Multiple septa detach from the epimysium and insert into both the overlying aponeurotic fascia and the underlying perimysial fascia.
- **Perimysial Fascia:** Surrounds bundles of muscle fibers within a muscle. It consists of connective tissue that penetrates the muscle to support and separate muscle fiber bundles (fascicles). This fascia provides the pathway for nerves and blood vessels to reach individual muscle fibers.
- **Endomysial Fascia:** Surrounds individual muscle fibers. It is a thin layer of connective tissue that supports capillaries and nerve fibers. The endomysium plays a crucial role in the transfer of force from the muscle fibers to the tendons.

3. Visceral Fascia (Subserous Fascia)

Location: Surrounds organs within the cavities of the body, such as the thoracic and abdominal cavities.

Composition: Thinner and more delicate than deep fascia, and often contains a larger amount of elastic fibers to accommodate the movement and expansion of organs.

Functions: The fascia holds organs in place and provides them with structural support. It also creates compartments within the body that can help limit the spread of infections or malignancies.

Each layer of fascia is integral to the functional architecture of the body, providing both structural support and flexibility. Problems in any layer of the fascia can lead to pain, reduced function, and mobility issues, highlighting the importance of this connective tissue system in overall health and well-being.

Functions of the Fascial System

The fascial system has several crucial functions:

1. **Support and Structure**: Fascia provides a supportive and stabilizing framework for all body structures. It holds organs in place and ensures that muscles and other structures maintain their proper alignment.
2. **Force Transmission**: Through its tensile strength and structural continuity, fascia transmits mechanical loads and muscle forces efficiently across the body. This helps in maintaining balance and coordination during movement.
3. **Protection**: Fascia acts as a protective layer over muscles and organs, cushioning them and reducing the impact of external forces.
4. **Separation and Compartmentalization**: By forming natural divisions between muscles and organs, fascia allows different body structures to slide smoothly over each other, facilitating efficient movement.

Fascial restrictions

Fascia restrictions, often simply referred to as fascial restrictions, occur when the fascia, the connective tissue that surrounds and supports all structures within the body, becomes tight, stiff, or forms adhesions. These restrictions can significantly impact the body's mobility, flexibility, and function. Here's an in-depth look at fascia restrictions:

Fascial restrictions refer to the tightening or stiffening of the fascia, the connective tissue that surrounds and supports muscles, bones, nerves, and organs throughout the body. Fascia is supposed to be flexible and able to stretch as you move. However, due to various factors such as injury, surgery, inflammation, poor posture, or lack of activity, the fascia can become restricted. When fascial restrictions occur, they can limit mobility and cause pain, discomfort, or decreased range of motion. These restrictions can have a cascading effect on the body, potentially affecting overall biomechanical efficiency and leading to compensations in movement, which in turn might cause further discomfort or injury.

Fascia Adhesion

Fascia adhesion occurs when the fascia, a thin layer of connective tissue that surrounds muscles, organs, and other structures, sticks to itself or to other tissues. This can restrict movement and cause pain.

Fascia Fibrosis

Fascia fibrosis is the thickening and stiffening of the fascia due to excessive collagen deposition, often as a response to chronic inflammation or injury. This condition is more severe than simple adhesions and can significantly impair function.

Causes of Fascia Restrictions

Fascia restrictions can arise from a variety of factors:

- **Injury**: Trauma from accidents or surgeries can lead to inflammation and subsequent fibrosis (scar tissue), which restricts the normal elasticity of fascia.
- **Repetitive Stress**: Repetitive activities or overuse injuries can lead to chronic inflammation and fibrotic changes in the fascia.
- **Poor Posture**: Prolonged poor posture can cause the fascia to adapt in maladaptive ways, leading to tension and restrictions.
- **Inactivity**: Lack of movement can cause fascia to become dehydrated and less pliable, making it prone to stiffness and adhesions.

- **Inflammatory Responses**: Systemic inflammation, as seen in various autoimmune disorders, can also affect the fascial system, making it less flexible.

Symptoms of Fascia Restrictions

The presence of fascial restrictions can manifest in various symptoms:

- **Reduced Mobility**: Stiffness and limited range of motion in joints.
- **Pain**: Chronic pain is often described as a deep, aching, or band-like pain that may increase with movement or touch.
- **Tension**: A feeling of tightness in the muscles and surrounding areas.
- **Sensory Changes**: Some individuals might experience tingling or numbness due to the pressure on nerves by tight fascia.
- **Misalignment**: Fascial restrictions can pull the body out of alignment, affecting posture and leading to compensatory patterns elsewhere in the body.

Ineffective Methods for Releasing Fascial Restrictions

The fascia system is so complex that it requires targeted tools to release each restricted layer. Random hand movements without gripping the fascia layer will not mobilize it to release the adhesions that cause the layers to stick together and prevent them from gliding freely on top of each other. An understanding of the physiology of the fascia system shows that certain approaches are ineffective for releasing it, including massage, foam rollers, manual therapy, Gua Sha, instrument-assisted soft tissue mobilization, stretching, and exercises.

1. **Foam rollers:** Typically, they provide only superficial pressure on the tissue. Gliding the foam roller over just the superficial layer will not release the adhesions, and the foam roller will not apply enough deep pressure to release the epimysium, perimysium, and endomysium layers.
2. **Deep tissue massage:** Involves the therapist using their hands, knuckles, and/or elbows to reach deeper layers of muscle. However, due to the width and diameter of the therapist's knuckles and elbows, it is difficult to

penetrate deep tissues and provide the consistent gripping forces necessary to release deep fascia adhesions.

3. **Manual therapy:** Similar to massage, it often involves using the knuckles, elbows, or hands to reach deeper tissues. However, the relatively large diameter of the therapist's hands and elbows may limit their ability to penetrate deeply enough to effect physiological changes in fascia layers located deep within muscles. Additionally, it is very difficult for the hand to grip deep fascia layers to release them.

4. **Exercises and stretching:** Do not exert sufficient mechanical force on fascia layers to cause adhesion release; they simply cause movement in the muscle.

5. **Myofascial release:** This involves applying gentle, sustained pressure to the superficial connective tissue, which addresses the superficial fascia layer but does not go deep enough to release the aponeurotic, epimysium,

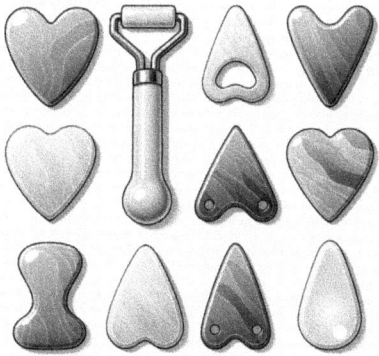

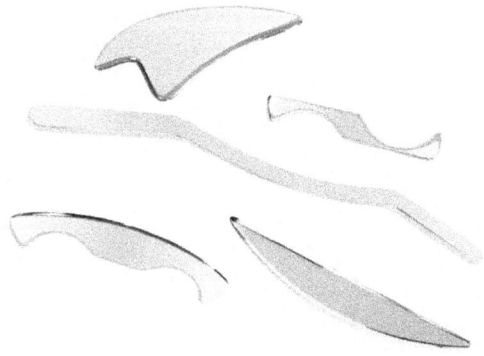

Instrument Assisted Soft Tissue Mobilization (IASTM)

Gua Sha

perimysium, and endomysium fascia layers.

6. **Gua Sha and Instrument-Assisted Soft Tissue Mobilization:** These techniques involve tools that might resemble rods or a butter knife, used to apply horizontal superficial force on the skin. Like manual therapy, they fail to penetrate deeply enough to alter the fascia system and are unable to grip the fascia layers to release them. This is like trying to unscrew a deep-set

screw in a car with a screwdriver that is too short; it simply cannot reach deep enough to be effective.

The Solution

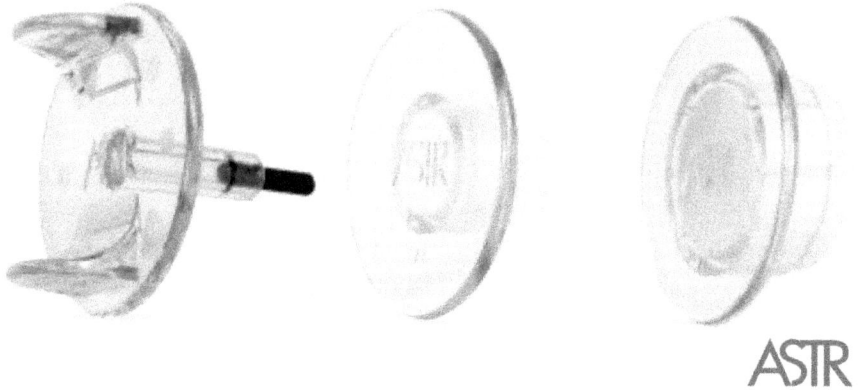

ASTR

Analyzing and testing current approaches that claim to provide myofascial release led me to realize that it is physiologically impossible to effectively target both superficial and deep fascia layers with these methods. This realization was the turning point that inspired the invention of ergonomically designed ASTR instruments. These instruments are specifically created to address superficial fascia, aponeurotic fascia, epimysium, perimysium, and endomysium layers. They are capable of penetrating up to 2 inches deep to release the epimysium, perimysium, and endomysium.

Summary

In cases of chronic conditions, the affected body part often remains caught in a relentless cycle, repeatedly fluctuating between inflammation and proliferation. This cycle results in significant inflammation and fibrosis, leading to muscle spasms and intense fascial restrictions. Nutritional deficiencies in vitamins and minerals may keep the body stuck in this cycle, blocking the progression to the maturation stage. Moreover, the presence of excessive fibrosis and intense fascial restrictions can further exacerbate the situation, making it more challenging to interrupt the ongoing cycle of chronic conditions.

This persistent issue underpins the biomedical model's inability to effectively treat chronic pain, as it primarily concentrates on symptoms rather than addressing underlying issues such as fibrotic tissue, fascial restrictions, and hormonal and nutritional imbalances.

Behavior Modification

Behavior modification is a therapeutic approach used to change undesirable behaviors into more desirable ones through the systematic application of learning principles and techniques. It's based on the theories of operant conditioning developed by John B. Watson and B.F. Skinner. The fundamental premise is that behaviors can be learned and unlearned based on the consequences they produce.

Behavior modification can be a valuable approach to addressing issues like poor posture, poor body mechanics, and the resultant pain. These behaviors, often developed over time through habits or environmental influences, can be altered using systematic techniques that encourage healthier patterns. Here's how behavior modification can be applied to these specific issues:

Identifying the Behaviors
The first step in the behavior modification process is to identify and clearly define the behaviors that need to be changed. For instance:

- **Poor Posture**: Slouching, leaning forward while sitting, or standing with an arched back.
- **Poor Body Mechanics**: Bending from the back instead of the knees to lift objects, or holding loads incorrectly.

Setting Goals
Set specific, measurable, achievable, relevant, and time-bound (SMART) goals for behavior change. For example:

- Improve sitting posture by taking a 5-minute break to walk around and take a break drinking water position every 20 minutes.
- Use correct lifting techniques for all lifting tasks throughout the workday.

Techniques for Behavior Modification
Several techniques can be employed to modify these behaviors:

1. **Education and Awareness**: Individuals often engage in poor habits due to a lack of awareness. Reading a book like this one on the importance of good posture and body mechanics, and their role in preventing pain, can be foundational.

2. **Self-Monitoring**: Monitor your own posture and mechanics. This could be done through diary keeping or setting reminders to check your posture.
3. **Positive Reinforcement**: Reward yourself or be rewarded for demonstrating good posture or proper lifting techniques. Rewards could be as simple as self-congratulation, a small treat, or recognition from a coworker.
4. **Cueing and Prompting**: Use visual or auditory cues to prompt the desired behavior. For instance, set up an ergonomic workstation that naturally encourages good posture, use apps or timers that remind you to adjust your posture regularly.
5. **Feedback**: Regular feedback from a coworker, spouse, or looking in the mirror can help you recognize when you lapse into poor habits and correct yourself.
6. **Modeling**: Demonstrating proper posture and body mechanics through workshops or video tutorials can provide a clear model for individuals to emulate. I have included posture training videos with this book; just scan the barcode below.

Maintenance and Generalization

Once new behaviors are learned, they need to be maintained and generalized to different settings. This can involve:

- **Consistent Practice**: Continuing to practice good posture and mechanics in all settings, not just at work or during specific tasks.
- **Social Support**: Encouraging family, friends, or colleagues to support and remind you about practicing good habits.
- **Adjusting Environments**: Modifying personal and professional environments to support these healthier behaviors permanently, like choosing chairs that support good posture or organizing workspaces to promote safe lifting practices.

Through these steps, behavior modification can effectively change harmful habits related to posture and body mechanics. This can reduce pain and improve overall health and well-being.

The Solution

Follow the recommendations in the 'Proper Posture and Body Mechanics' chapter to correct potential bad ergonomics that may exacerbate your symptoms. For complex conditions where symptoms persist even after correcting body posture and ergonomics, it is advisable to seek help from a healthcare provider trained in ergonomics and behavior modifications.

A behavioral and ergonomic therapist, trained in evaluating a patient's body posture, body mechanics, and condition-specific habits, should assess your condition to determine the necessary behavioral modifications. For example, common poor habits like chewing gum, which are associated with jaw pain, need to be changed to minimize the risk of re-injuring the jaw.

Vitamin, Mineral, and Hormonal Imbalances

The human body requires 13 vitamins and 16 minerals to function optimally, many of which are essential for hormone and neurotransmitter production. Since the body cannot synthesize these nutrients, they must be obtained through diet and/or supplements. Deficiencies in certain vitamins can contribute to muscle and joint pain, as these nutrients are vital for maintaining bone health, muscle function, and overall musculoskeletal integrity. Deficiencies in vitamins and minerals can cause the body to remain stuck in the inflammation-proliferation cycle, preventing progression to the maturation stage. Addressing these deficiencies can help alleviate symptoms and enhance joint and muscle health. Key vitamins linked to muscle and joint pain include:

1. Vitamin D
- **Role**: Vitamin D is essential for calcium absorption in the gut and maintains adequate serum calcium and phosphate concentrations to enable normal mineralization of bone. It is also necessary for bone growth and bone remodeling by osteoblasts and osteoclasts.
- **Deficiency Symptoms:** Deficiency can lead to bone-softening diseases such as rickets in children and osteomalacia in adults. It is also associated with osteoporosis and an increased risk of fractures. Muscle weakness and pain are common symptoms of vitamin D deficiency.
- **Sources:** Sun exposure, fatty fish, and supplements.
- Optimal dosing requires lab-guided monitoring, as excessive vitamin D may lead to hypercalcemia, kidney strain, and increased cardiovascular risk.

2. Vitamin C
- **Role**: Role: Vitamin C is important for the synthesis of collagen, an essential component of connective tissues in the body, found in the skin, tendons, ligaments, and bones.
- **Deficiency Symptoms:** Severe vitamin C deficiency leads to scurvy, which manifests with symptoms like joint pain and swelling, muscle aches, and weakness due to the weakening of connective tissues.
- **Sources:** Citrus fruits, strawberries, kiwis, bell peppers, and green vegetables.

3. Vitamin B12

- **Role:** Vitamin B12 is vital for nerve function and the formation of red blood cells. It is also important for DNA synthesis and maintaining healthy nerve cells.
- **Deficiency Symptoms:** B12 deficiency can cause fatigue, weakness, nerve damage, and neurological problems, which may manifest as numbness and tingling in the hands and feet. Some people may experience muscle weakness and joint pain as indirect symptoms of nerve damage.
- **Sources:** Meat, dairy products, and eggs.
- Excessive intake may cause numbness, burning sensations, and itching, emphasizing the need for personalized dosing.

4. Vitamin B1 (Thiamine)

- **Role**: Thiamine plays a crucial role in the metabolism of carbohydrates, helping turn nutrients into energy essential for nerve, muscle, and heart function.
- **Deficiency Symptoms**: Deficiency can lead to beriberi, which includes symptoms such as muscle weakness, pain, and peripheral neuropathy.
- **Sources**: Whole grains, pork, and legumes.

5. Vitamin E

- **Role:** Vitamin E has antioxidant properties that protect cells from oxidative stress. It also helps maintain muscle and immune system health.
- **Deficiency Symptoms:** Vitamin E deficiency can cause neuromuscular problems, including muscle weakness and limb and joint pain.
- **Sources:** Nuts, seeds, and green leafy vegetables.

Muscle and joint pain can be exacerbated by deficiencies in certain minerals that are vital for muscular function, nerve signaling, and bone health. Here are some critical minerals whose deficiencies might lead to such symptoms:

Vitamin, Mineral, and Hormonal Imbalances

1. Magnesium

- **Role:** Magnesium is essential for over 300 enzyme reactions in the body, including those involved in the contraction and relaxation of muscles and nerve function.
- **Deficiency Symptoms:** Symptoms of magnesium deficiency include muscle cramps, spasms, and widespread muscle pain, often referred to as fibromyalgia. Magnesium deficiency can also lead to increased inflammation, which could exacerbate joint pain.
- **Sources:** Leafy green vegetables, nuts, seeds, and whole grains.
- Excessive intake may cause gastrointestinal symptoms, confusion, cardiac arrest, and kidney dysfunction, emphasizing the need for personalized dosing.

2. Calcium

- **Role:** Calcium is crucial for maintaining strong bones and the proper function of nerves and muscles.
- **Deficiency Symptoms:** Inadequate calcium can lead to osteopenia and osteoporosis, increasing the risk of fractures and causing bone pain. It may also cause muscle aches and spasms.
- **Sources:** Dairy products and leafy greens.

3. Potassium

- **Role**: Potassium is important for muscle and nerve cell function. It helps regulate heartbeat and muscle function.
- **Deficiency Symptoms**: Deficiency in potassium (hypokalemia) can result in muscle weakness, cramps, stiffness, and joint pain. Severe deficiency can be life-threatening.
- **Sources**: Bananas, oranges, cantaloupe, honeydew, apricots, grapefruit (some are also sources of beta-carotene), cooked spinach, cooked broccoli, potatoes, sweet potatoes, mushrooms, peas, cucumbers, zucchini, eggplant, pumpkins, and leafy greens.
- Potassium overload may also cause kidney dysfunction and impair neuromuscular function. For this reason, laboratory testing of serum potassium and kidney function is essential before initiating

supplementation. Proper assessment ensures that potassium levels are corrected safely and effectively without placing additional strain on vital organs.

4. Iron
- **Role**: Iron is crucial for the production of hemoglobin, a protein in red blood cells that helps carry oxygen to tissues, including muscles, which is vital for their function and repair.
- **Deficiency Symptoms**: Iron deficiency can cause anemia, leading to fatigue, weakness, and pale skin. While not directly causing joint pain, the lack of oxygen can increase muscle fatigue and soreness.
- **Sources**: Red meat, poultry, fish, legumes, and dark leafy greens.
- Excessive iron supplementation can promote oxidative stress, joint pain, liver dysfunction, and heart failure, so individualized dosing is critical.

5. Zinc
- **Role**: Zinc plays a role in cell division, cell growth, wound healing, and the breakdown of carbohydrates. Zinc is also necessary for the senses of smell and taste.
- **Deficiency Symptoms**: Zinc deficiency can lead to a weakened immune response, slow wound healing, and can indirectly contribute to muscle and joint pain through weakened immune and inflammatory responses.
- **Sources**: Meat, shellfish, legumes, seeds, nuts, dairy products, eggs, and whole grains.
- Supplementation should be carefully monitored, as excessive zinc can lead to copper depletion and hormonal imbalances.

If you're experiencing persistent muscle and joint pain, it may be worth investigating whether a mineral deficiency could be a contributing factor. However, it's important to seek advice from healthcare professionals trained in nutrition evaluation for proper diagnosis and treatment, which may include dietary changes or supplementation.

Hormonal imbalances can significantly impact muscle and joint health, leading to discomfort and pain. Several hormones, if not balanced correctly, can contribute to or exacerbate these symptoms. Here's how specific hormonal imbalances can cause muscle and joint pain:

1. Estrogen
- **Role:** Estrogen helps to regulate fluids in the body and maintains the health of joints by influencing collagen production and preserving bone strength.
- **Imbalance Effects:** Low estrogen levels, particularly common during menopause or as a result of certain treatments like aromatase inhibitors for breast cancer, can lead to joint pain, stiffness, and an increased risk of osteoporosis. Estrogen's anti-inflammatory effects are reduced when levels drop, potentially increasing inflammation around joints.

2. Cortisol
- **Role:** Cortisol, known as the "stress hormone," helps regulate the body's response to stress. It has natural anti-inflammatory effects and influences energy production in muscles.
- **Imbalance Effects:** Chronic stress, leading to prolonged high cortisol levels, can eventually cause the hormone's production to falter. Low cortisol (as seen in adrenal insufficiency) can cause joint pain and muscle aches, while consistently high levels can lead to muscle weakness and chronic joint inflammation.

3. Thyroid Hormones
- **Role**: Thyroid hormones regulate metabolism, energy generation, and overall physiological balance.
- **Imbalance Effects**: Both hyperthyroidism (excess thyroid hormone) and hypothyroidism (insufficient thyroid hormone) can lead to joint and muscle pain. Hypothyroidism is particularly known for causing muscle weakness, stiffness, aches, and tenderness.

4. Parathyroid Hormone

- **Role**: Parathyroid hormone helps regulate calcium levels in the blood, which is essential for nerve and muscle function.
- **Imbalance Effects**: Overactivity of the parathyroid glands (hyperparathyroidism) can lead to too much calcium in the blood, weakening bones and causing bone and joint pain.

5. Testosterone

- **Role:** Testosterone is important for muscle mass and strength, as well as bone density.
- **Imbalance Effects:** Low testosterone levels can lead to a decrease in muscle mass and strength, which can exacerbate joint pain due to less support around the joint structures. It also affects bone density, potentially leading to osteoporosis.

6. Growth Hormone

- **Role**: Growth hormone plays a key role in muscle and bone growth and maintenance.
- **Imbalance Effects**: Deficiency can lead to a decrease in muscle mass and bone density, increasing the risk of joint and muscle pain.

Addressing Hormonal Imbalances

If you suspect that a hormonal imbalance is contributing to muscle and joint pain, it's essential to consult with a healthcare provider. They can diagnose hormonal imbalances through blood tests and recommend appropriate treatments, such as hormone replacement therapy, lifestyle changes, and possibly dietary adjustments. Managing stress, ensuring adequate sleep, engaging in regular physical activity, and maintaining a balanced diet can also help maintain hormonal balance and reduce symptoms.

Biomedical Model's Shortcomings

Unfortunately, our healthcare system often lacks proper nutrition education for medical doctors. This was one of the reasons I went from one doctor to another without receiving adequate help. They failed to evaluate my diet or direct me to nutrition-focused labs that could identify the root causes of my health issues. I've had conversations with many doctors across different disciplines who expressed concerns about the biomedical model's shortcomings, particularly the lack of nutrition education in medical schools and the subsequent inability to evaluate patients' nutritional deficiencies effectively.

Before studying nutrition, I spent thousands on supplements without seeing improvement. I often assumed I had deficiencies related to the benefits of various vitamins and minerals I read about. Sometimes my assumptions were correct, but frequently I took unnecessary supplements, which led to overdosing and adverse effects. I advise against this approach due to its potential risks. After educating myself and conducting proper evaluations of my vitamin, mineral, and hormone levels, I could finally pinpoint the root causes of my chronic pain, fatigue, and migraines, eliminating years of guesswork.

Case Study 9: Knees Pain

I had a patient who came to the clinic with bilateral knee pain and was wheelchair-bound, unable to walk due to her pain. During her evaluation, she mentioned not having bowel movements for two weeks, being diabetic, and not consuming protein and fiber for a while. Although she presented with knee pain, her history suggested several nutritional deficiencies and an imbalanced diet. If I had only followed the physical therapy model, I would have provided modalities for pain and exercises to strengthen her knees. Instead, I used the BPS model and provided dietary, lab, and supplementation recommendations. Two weeks later, the patient returned to the clinic walking and without knee pain, as her issue was primarily due to malnutrition.

The solution

If you are experiencing chronic muscle and joint pain, there is a high likelihood that you are suffering from various vitamin and mineral deficiencies, as well as hormonal imbalances, which can slow down your normal healing cycle or trap your body in a vicious cycle of inflammation and proliferation. It's important to consult a healthcare provider trained to release fibrotic tissue and fascia restrictions, as well as properly evaluate nutritional deficiencies and interpret lab results for vitamins, minerals, and hormones. When seeking healthcare providers in this area, look for someone who has studied nutrition and understands how to properly evaluate imbalances in vitamins, minerals, and hormones.

Conclusion

Conclusion

Our healthcare system often lacks proper nutrition education for medical doctors. This was one of the reasons I went from one doctor to another without receiving adequate help. They failed to evaluate my diet or direct me to nutrition-focused labs that could identify the root causes of my health issues. I've had conversations with many doctors across different disciplines who expressed concerns about the biomedical model's shortcomings, particularly the lack of nutrition education in medical schools and the subsequent inability to evaluate patients' nutritional deficiencies effectively.

Based on an overwhelming number of studies, the following treatments have demonstrated either short-term pain reduction or no pain reduction for musculoskeletal pain. In some cases, the placebo effect performed better than the biomedical model due to the severe adverse effects of the biomedical model treatments. Here is the list of ineffective treatments for chronic pain:

1. Opioids
2. Non-steroidal Anti-inflammatory Drugs (NSAIDs)
3. Stretching and Exercises
4. Massage Therapy
5. Acupuncture
6. Steroid injections
7. Trigger Point Injection
8. Dry Needle
9. Therapeutic Ultrasound
10. Electrical Stimulation
11. Platelet-Rich Plasma (PRP)
12. Manual Therapy - Soft Tissue Mobilization
13. Instrument Assisted Soft Tissue Mobilization (IASTM)
14. Myofascial Release
15. Joint Manipulation - Joint Mobilization
16. Manual Therapy and Exercise
17. Kinesio Taping
18. Active Release Technique (ART)
19. Strain Counterstrain Technique (SCS)

Conclusion

20. Craniosacral Therapy
21. McKenzie Method

Overwhelming research studies have confirmed the efficacy of the BPS model in relieving chronic pain, improving quality of life, and transitioning patients back to normal activities. It is more cost-effective and time-efficient when the BPS model is provided by a single healthcare provider. This approach not only improves patient outcomes and experiences but also increases job satisfaction among healthcare providers.

When the BPS model is implemented by a single healthcare provider, it offers several benefits. It reduces healthcare costs by consolidating multiple specialists' roles, streamlines care by avoiding the need for multiple visits, and improves outcomes through a comprehensive understanding of the patient's health. This approach enhances the patient experience by fostering a stronger provider-patient relationship, leading to better treatment compliance and satisfaction. Additionally, it allows for comprehensive health management by addressing various factors simultaneously and increases provider satisfaction by enabling them to see the full impact of their care. Implementing the BPS model in this way provides a more personalized, efficient, and effective healthcare experience for both patients and providers.

I encourage you to implement the following important parts of the BPS model at home: posture and body mechanics training, stress management, behavior modification, and an anti-inflammatory diet. These could relieve your symptoms when you follow the instructions in the designated chapters of this book.
In cases of chronic conditions, the affected body part often remains caught in a relentless cycle, repeatedly fluctuating between inflammation and proliferation. This cycle results in significant inflammation and fibrosis, leading to muscle spasms and intense fascial restrictions. Nutritional deficiencies in vitamins and minerals may keep the body stuck in this cycle, blocking the progression to the maturation stage. Moreover, excessive fibrosis and intense fascial restrictions can further exacerbate the situation, making it more challenging to interrupt the ongoing cycle of chronic conditions. This persistent issue underpins the

Conclusion

biomedical model's inability to effectively treat chronic pain, as it primarily concentrates on symptoms rather than addressing underlying issues such as fibrotic tissue, fascial restrictions, and hormonal and nutritional imbalances.

If you are experiencing chronic muscle and joint pain, there's a high likelihood that you are suffering from various vitamin and mineral deficiencies, as well as hormonal imbalances, which can slow down your normal healing cycle or trap your body in a vicious cycle of inflammation and proliferation. It's important to consult a healthcare provider trained to release fibrotic tissue and fascia restrictions, as well as properly evaluate nutritional deficiencies and interpret lab results for vitamins, minerals, and hormones. When seeking healthcare providers in this area, look for someone who has studied nutrition and understands how to properly evaluate imbalances in vitamins, minerals, and hormones.

Recommended Resources

How to Access Online Content

1. Open the camera app on your smartphone.
2. Point the camera at the barcode.
3. A notification will appear with a link. Tap the notification to open the link in your browser.

1. Posture and Body Mechanics Training Videos

2. Case Studies and Recorded Live Treatment Videos

3. <u>Limited Time Offer</u>: FREE 30-minute Health Coach Consultation

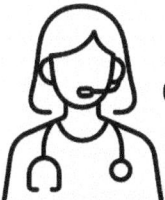

FREE
CONSULTATION
WITH
HEALTH COACH

GET STARTED

EAT TO HEAL

The ASTR Diet: Unlock the Healing Power of Food to End Sickness and Thrive

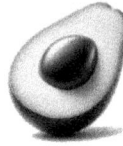

- Achieve Lasting Weight Loss
- Reverse Chronic Diseases Naturally
- Heal Inflammation and Pain
- Boost Energy and Vitality
- 3 Steps to Transform Your Health

Dr. Joseph Jacobs, DPT, ACN

BEATING ANXIETY & DEPRESSION

BONUS VIDEOS

14 NATURAL SECRETS TO A HAPPIER LIFE

- Conquer Anxiety & Depression Naturally
- Heal the Root Causes & Reclaim Your Life
- Created by a Doctor Who Conquered PTSD & Depression
- Science-Based Strategies for Lasting Change

Dr. Joseph Jacobs, DPT, ACN

BEATING
MIGRAINES

BONUS VIDEOS

7 NATURAL SECRETS FOR
LASTING RELIEF

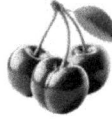

- End Migraines Naturally
- Clinically Proven Methods
- Treat the Root Cause, Not Symptoms
- Insights from a Doctor & Migraine Survivor
- Research-Backed Relief for Life

Dr. Joseph Jacobs, DPT, ACN

BEATING
BACK PAIN

BONUS VIDEOS

7 NATURAL SECRETS FOR
LASTING RELIEF

- End Back Pain Naturally
- Clinically Tested, Doctor-Approved
- Fix the Root Causes, Not Just Symptoms
- Backed by Science & Research
- Created by a Doctor Who Beat Chronic Pain

Dr. Joseph Jacobs, DPT, ACN

REVERSING
HIGH BLOOD
PRESSURE

**7 NATURAL SECRETS TO SAFELY
LOWER BLOOD PRESSURE**

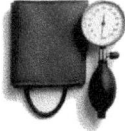

- Natural Solutions That Work
- Backed by Extensive Research
- Fix the Root Cause, Not Just the Numbers
- No Drugs, No Side Effects

Dr. Joseph Jacobs, DPT, ACN

REVERSING
DIABETES

**10 NATURAL SECRETS TO REVERSE
DIABETES WITHOUT DRUGS**

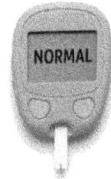

NORMAL

- Drug-Free, Side-Effect-Free, Science-Backed Healing
- Treat the Root Cause, Not Just the Symptoms
- Proven Natural Strategies That Get Results

Dr. Joseph Jacobs, DPT, ACN

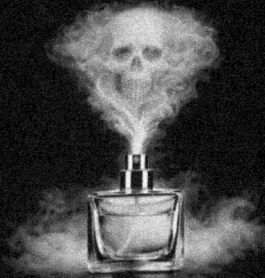

KILLED BY
FRAGRANCE

How Synthetic Scents Make Us Sick

- Exposed by peer-reviewed research
- Links everyday fragrance exposure to chronic disease
- Built on science, not opinion

Dr. Joseph Jacobs, DPT, ACN

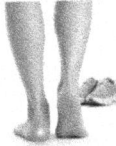

Your
SHOES
HURT YOU
Why Does Your Pain Keep Coming
Back and *How to Fix It*

BONUS VIDEOS

- Fix Your Feet. Fix Your Pain.
- Why Modern Shoes Create Chronic Pain
- Backed by Biomechanics and Clinical Research

Dr. Joseph Jacobs, DPT, ACN

Glossary

Aesthetic: Pertaining to the appreciation of beauty or good taste.

Acupuncture: A traditional Chinese medicine technique involving the insertion of thin needles into specific points on the body to alleviate pain and treat various health conditions.

Adaptability: The ability of an organism to adjust to changes in its environment or to changes in itself.

Angiogenesis: The formation of new blood vessels.

Anemia: A condition in which the blood doesn't have enough healthy red blood cells.

Appendectomy: Surgical removal of the appendix.

Aponeurotic Fascia: Dense connective tissue that connects muscle to muscle or muscle to bone.

Arthritis: Inflammation of one or more joints, causing pain and stiffness.

Aortic Aneurysm Repair: Surgical procedure to fix a weakened and bulging section of the aorta.

Autoimmune: Pertaining to the immune response of an organism against its own healthy cells and tissues.

Behavior Modification: Techniques used to change maladaptive behaviors and reinforce desirable behaviors.

Beriberi: A disease caused by a deficiency of thiamine (vitamin B1).

Biological: Relating to biology or living organisms.

Biomedical Model: A perspective that explains illness solely in terms of biological factors.

Biopsychosocial: An approach that considers biological, psychological, and social factors in health and illness.

Blood Pressure: The pressure of circulating blood against the walls of blood vessels.

Bursitis: Inflammation of the bursae (small fluid-filled sacs) that cushion the bones, tendons, and muscles near joints.

Capillaries: The smallest blood vessels where the exchange of water, oxygen, carbon dioxide, and many other nutrients and waste substances occurs between blood and surrounding tissues.

Carpal Tunnel: A narrow passageway in the wrist through which nerves and tendons pass.

Glossary

Carpal Tunnel Syndrome: A condition caused by compression of the median nerve as it travels through the carpal tunnel, leading to pain, numbness, and tingling in the hand and arm.

Cardiovascular: Pertaining to the heart and blood vessels.

Cohort Studies: A type of observational study that follows a group of people over time to determine how certain exposures affect the incidence of a particular outcome.

Collagen: The main structural protein found in skin and other connective tissues.

Coronary Artery Bypass Grafting (CABG) Surgery: A procedure to improve blood flow to the heart by diverting blood around blocked or narrowed coronary arteries.

Contraction: The process in which a muscle becomes shorter and tighter.

Cortisol: A steroid hormone produced by the adrenal glands, often released in response to stress.

Craniotomy: Surgical removal of part of the bone from the skull to expose the brain.

Craniosacral Therapy: A gentle, hands-on approach that releases tensions deep in the body to relieve pain and dysfunction.

Cross-Sectional Studies: Studies that analyze data from a population at a specific point in time.

Cytokines: Small proteins that are crucial in controlling the growth and activity of other immune system cells and blood cells.

Depression: A mood disorder causing a persistent feeling of sadness and loss of interest.

Destruction Stage: The phase in tissue injury where damaged cells and tissues are broken down and removed.

Diabetes: A group of diseases that result in too much sugar in the blood.

Disease: A disorder of structure or function in a human, animal, or plant.

DNA: Deoxyribonucleic acid, the carrier of genetic information.

Dry Needling: A technique used by physical therapists and other healthcare practitioners to treat myofascial pain by inserting fine needles into trigger points.

Electrical Stimulation: The use of electrical impulses to stimulate nerves and muscles.

Glossary

Elastin: A protein that provides elasticity to tissues and organs.

Endomysial Fascia: Connective tissue surrounding individual muscle fibers.

Endomysium: The connective tissue that wraps each individual muscle fiber.

Endomysium Fascia: Connective tissue surrounding each individual muscle fiber.

Engulf Bacteria: The process by which phagocytes (white blood cells) ingest or engulf bacteria to eliminate them.

Epimysial Fascia: The connective tissue sheath that surrounds an entire muscle.

Epimysium: The connective tissue surrounding an entire muscle.

Epimysium Fascia: Connective tissue surrounding an entire muscle.

Evidence-Based Practice: Healthcare practices based on scientific evidence to achieve the best outcomes for patients.

Fascia: A band or sheet of connective tissue, primarily collagen, that supports and surrounds muscles and other organs.

Fascia System: The network of connective tissues, including fasciae, that support and connect all parts of the body.

Fascicles: Bundles of skeletal muscle fibers surrounded by perimysium.

Fasical Restriction: Limited movement or mobility due to tightness or adhesions in the fascia.

Fibroblast: A cell that produces collagen and other fibers.

Fibronectin: A glycoprotein that helps cells attach to the extracellular matrix.

Fibrosis: The thickening and scarring of connective tissue, usually as a result of injury.

Fibrotic Tissue: Tissue that has undergone fibrosis, becoming thickened and scarred.

Fibromyalgia: A disorder characterized by widespread musculoskeletal pain accompanied by fatigue, sleep, memory, and mood issues.

Fructose: A simple sugar found in many plants.

Frozen Shoulder: A condition characterized by stiffness and pain in the shoulder joint.

Gastrointestinal: Pertaining to the stomach and intestines.

Growth Hormone: A hormone that stimulates growth, cell reproduction, and cell regeneration.

Glossary

Gua Sha: A traditional East Asian healing technique involving scraping of the skin with a massage tool to improve circulation.

Heart Attack: A condition where blood flow to the heart is blocked, causing tissue damage.

Hemoglobin: A protein in red blood cells that carries oxygen throughout the body.

Hemorrhage: An escape of blood from a ruptured blood vessel.

Hydrogen: The chemical element with the symbol H and atomic number 1.

Hypokalemia: A condition where blood's potassium levels are too low.

Inflammation: A protective response involving immune cells, blood vessels, and molecular mediators to eliminate the initial cause of cell injury, clear out damaged cells, and establish repair.

Inflammation Stage: The initial phase of the healing process, where the body's immune response is activated to remove harmful stimuli.

Instrument-Assisted Soft Tissue Mobilization: A manual therapy technique where instruments are used to manipulate the skin, myofascia, and muscles.

Instrument Assisted Soft Tissue Mobilization (IASTM): A technique where instruments are used to help break down scar tissue and fascial restrictions.

Insomnia: Persistent difficulty in falling or staying asleep.

Insulin Resistance: A condition where cells in the body become less responsive to insulin, leading to elevated blood sugar levels.

Joint Manipulation: A technique where a therapist uses their hands to apply controlled force to a joint.

Joint Mobilization: A manual therapy technique to improve joint function and range of motion.

Joint Mobilization or Manipulation: Techniques to restore the motion and function of joints.

Kinesio Taping: A therapeutic taping technique used to support and stabilize muscles and joints without restricting their range of motion.

Ligaments: Tough, elastic bands of connective tissue that connect bones to other bones.

Margarine: A spread used for flavoring, baking, and cooking, made from vegetable oils.

Glossary

Manual Therapy: Hands-on techniques used by therapists to manipulate the muscles, joints, and soft tissues of the body.

Maturation Stage: The final phase of wound healing, where the tissue gains strength and flexibility.

McKenzie Method: A treatment approach for spinal and extremity pain developed by physical therapist Robin McKenzie.

Meta-analysis: A statistical analysis that combines the results of multiple scientific studies.

Metabolic: Relating to metabolism, the chemical processes that occur within a living organism to maintain life.

Migraines: A type of headache characterized by severe, throbbing pain, usually on one side of the head.

Mindfulness: The practice of being aware and present in the moment without judgment.

Mineralization: The process where minerals are deposited in the body, particularly in bones and teeth.

Musculoskeletal: Pertaining to the muscles and the skeleton.

Myofascial: Relating to or involving the fascia surrounding and separating muscle tissue.

Myofascial Release: A manual therapy technique that involves applying gentle sustained pressure into the myofascial connective tissue restrictions.

Myogenesis: The formation and development of muscle tissue.

Neurological: Relating to the nervous system.

Neuromuscular: Pertaining to both nerves and muscles.

Neuromuscular: Involving both nerves and muscles.

Neurotransmitter: Chemicals that transmit signals across a synapse from one neuron to another.

NSAIDs: Nonsteroidal anti-inflammatory drugs, a class of medications used to reduce inflammation and pain.

Observational Studies: Studies that observe outcomes without intervention by the researcher.

Opioids: A class of drugs used to reduce pain but can also cause addiction.

Osteoblasts: Cells that synthesize bone.

Osteopenia: A condition where bone mineral density is lower than normal.

Glossary

Osteoporosis: A condition characterized by weak and brittle bones.

Pathogens: Microorganisms that cause disease.

Parathyroid: Glands located in the neck that regulate calcium levels in the blood.

Phagocytic: Relating to phagocytes, cells that engulf and absorb bacteria and other small cells and particles.

Phagocytic: Relating to the process by which cells ingest and eliminate particles.

Plantar Fasciitis: Inflammation of the plantar fascia, the thick band of tissue that runs across the bottom of the foot.

Platelet-Rich Plasma (PRP): A treatment that uses a concentration of platelets from the patient's own blood to accelerate the healing of injured tendons, ligaments, muscles, and joints.

Proliferation Stage: The phase of wound healing where new tissue and blood vessels form.

Psychological: Relating to the mind or mental processes.

Radiation: The emission of energy as electromagnetic waves or as moving subatomic particles, especially high-energy particles that cause ionization.

Remodeling Phase: The final stage of tissue repair where collagen is remodeled, and the tissue matures.

Sciatica: Pain affecting the back, hip, and outer side of the leg, caused by compression of a spinal nerve root in the lower back.

Soft Tissue Mobilization: A manual therapy technique to break up inelastic or fibrous muscle tissue, move tissue fluids, and relax muscle tension.

Steroid Injections: Injections of corticosteroids to reduce inflammation and provide pain relief.

Strain Counterstrain Technique (SCS): A manual therapy technique used to relieve muscle and connective tissue tightness by placing the body in a position of comfort.

Stroke: A medical condition where poor blood flow to the brain results in cell death.

Subcutaneous: Situated or applied under the skin.

Superficial Fascia: The lowermost layer of the skin that contains fat and connective tissue.

Glossary

Superficial Fascia: Connective tissue beneath the skin that encloses, stabilizes, and separates muscles and internal organs.

Systematic Review: A research method that involves systematically searching for, appraising, and synthesizing research evidence.

Tendon: A flexible but inelastic cord of strong fibrous collagen tissue attaching a muscle to a bone.

Tendonitis: Inflammation of a tendon.

Testosterone: The primary male sex hormone responsible for the development of male reproductive tissues and secondary sexual characteristics.

Thyroid: A gland in the neck that secretes hormones regulating growth and development through the rate of metabolism.

Trigger Point: A sensitive area in the muscle or connective tissue that becomes painful when compressed.

Trigger Point Injection: An injection into a trigger point to relieve pain and improve function.

Ultrasound Therapy: A treatment that uses high-frequency sound waves to promote tissue healing and reduce pain.

Ubiquity: The state of being everywhere or in many places simultaneously.

Vascularity: The degree to which blood vessels are present in tissue.

References

1. Joseph J, Madison S, Tiffany J, Henry H, Mario V, et al . Evaluating the Effectiveness of Treatment Options for Pain: Literature Review.Ortho Res Online J. 3(5). OPROJ.000574.2018. DOI: 10.31031/OPROJ.2018.03.000574

2. University of Rochester Medical Center. (n.d.). The Biopsychosocial Approach. Retrieved from https://www.urmc.rochester.edu/medialibraries/urmcmedia/education/md/documents/biopsychosocial-model-approach.pdfhttps://www.cdc.gov/nchs/fastats/diseases-and-conditions.htm

3. Yaribeygi, H., Panahi, Y., Sahraei, H., Johnston, T. P., & Sahebkar, A. (2017). The impact of stress on body function: A review. EXCLI journal, 16, 1057-1072.https://www.merriam-webster.com/dictionary/disease

4. Engel GL: The need for a new medical model: a challenge for biomedicine. Science 1977;196:129-136.

5. Engel GL: The clinical application of the biopsychosocial model. Am J Psychiatry 1980;137:535-544. https://pubmed.ncbi.nlm.nih.gov/847460/

6. Frankel RM, Quill TE, McDaniel SH (Eds.): The Biopsychosocial Approach: Past, Present, Future.University of Rochester Press, Rochester, NY, 2003.

7. Borrell-Carrió F, Suchman AL, Epstein RM: The biopsychosocial model 25 years later: principles, practice, and scientific inquiry. Ann Fam Med 2004;2:576-582.

8. Cohen J, Brown Clark S: John Romano and George Engel: Their Lives and Work.University of Rochester Press, Rochester, NY, and Boydell and Brewer Limited, Suffolk UK, 2010.

9. Challenging Traditional Perspectives on Pain Relief | Dr. Jacobs TEDx Talk

10. Hannah K. Scott, Ankit Jain, Mark Cogburn: Behavior Modification. Treasure Island (FL): StatPearls Publishing; 2024 Jan. 2023 Jul 10.https://pubmed.ncbi.nlm.nih.gov/29083709/

11. Straube, S., Andrew Moore, R., Derry, S., & McQuay, H. J. (2010). Vitamin D and chronic pain. Pain, 149(1), 14-19. https://www.ncbi.nlm.nih.gov/pmc/articles/PMC4427945/

12. https://www.betterhealth.vic.gov.au/health/healthyliving/Vitamins-and-minerals

13. Tzenalis A, Beneka A, Malliou P, Godolias, G, Staurou N. The biopsychosocial treatment approach for chronic neck and back pain: A systematic review of randomized controlled trials. European Psychomotricity Journal. 2016; 8: 29-48.

14. Beardsley C, Škarabot J. Effects of self-myofascial release: A systematic review. Journal of Bodywork and Movement Therapies. 2015;19(4):747-758. doi:10.1016/j.jbmt.2015.08.007.

15. Reuben DB, Alvanzo AA, Ashikaga T, et al. National Institutes of Health Pathways to Prevention Workshop: The Role of Opioids in the Treatment of Chronic Pain. Annals of Internal Medicine. 2015;162(4):295-300. doi:10.7326/m14-2775.

16. ASAM Opioid Addiction 2016 Facts & Figures. American Society of Addiction Medicine

17. Prescription opioids and heroin epidemic in Georgia. Substance Abuse Research Alliance (SARA) | Georgia Prevention Project. 2017.

18. Bervoets DC, Luijsterburg PA, Alessie JJ, Buijs MJ, Verhagen AP. Massage therapy has short-term benefits for people with common musculoskeletal disorders compared to no treatment: a systematic review. Journal of Physiotherapy. 2015;61(3):106-116. doi:10.1016/j.jphys.2015.05.018.

19. Chou R, Deyo R, Friedly J, et al. Nonpharmacologic Therapies for Low Back Pain. Annals of Internal Medicine. 2017;167(8):493-505. doi:10.7326/l17-0395.

References

20. Miller J, Gross A, Dsylva J, et al. Manual therapy and exercise for neck pain: A systematic review. Manual Therapy. 2010;15(4):334-354. doi:10.1016/j.math.2010.02.007.
21. Cheatham SW, Lee M, Cain M, et al. : The efficacy of instrument assisted soft tissue mobilization: a systematic review. J Can Chiropr Assoc, 2016, 60: 200–211.
22. ngel G. The need for a new medical model: a challenge for biomedicine. Science. 1977;196(4286):129-136. doi:10.1126/science.847460.
23. Shete K, Suryawanshi P, Gandhi N. Management of low back pain in computer users: A multidisciplinary approach. Journal of Craniovertebral Junction and Spine. 2012;3(1):7-10. doi:10.4103/0974-8237.110117.
24. Kamper SJ, Apeldoorn AT, Chiarotto A, et al. Multidisciplinary biopsychosocial rehabilitation for chronic low back pain: Cochrane systematic review and meta-analysis. Bmj. 2015;350. doi:10.1136/bmj.h444.
25. Guzmán J, Esmail R, Karjalainen K, Malmivaara A Irvin E, Bombardier C et al. Multidisciplinary rehabilitation for chronic low back pain: systematic review BMJ 2001; 322 :1511-1516. doi:10.1136/bmj.322.7301.1511.
26. Korff MRV. Long-term use of opioids for complex chronic pain. Best Practice & Research Clinical Rheumatology. 2013;27(5):663-672. doi:10.1016/j.berh.2013.09.011.
27. Machado GC, Maher CG, Ferreira PH, Day RO, Pinheiro MB, Ferreira ML. Non-steroidal anti-inflammatory drugs for spinal pain: a systematic review and meta-analysis. Annals of the Rheumatic Diseases. 2017;76(7):1269-1278. doi:10.1136/annrheumdis-2016-210597.
28. Varas-Lorenzo C, Riera-Guardia N, Calingaert B, et al. Stroke risk and NSAIDs: a systematic review of observational studies. Pharmacoepidemiology and Drug Safety. 2011;20(12):1225-1236. doi:10.1002/pds.2227.
29. Turk DC, Okifuji A. Treatment of Chronic Pain Patients: Clinical Outcomes, Cost-Effectiveness, and Cost-Benefits of Multidisciplinary Pain Centers. Critical Reviews in Physical and Rehabilitation Medicine. 1998;10(2):181-208. doi:10.1615/critrevphysrehabilmed.v10.i2.40.
30. Mavrocordatos et al. Benefits of the multidisciplinary team for the patient
31. Espejo-Antúnez L, Tejeda JF-H, Albornoz-Cabello M, et al. Dry needling in the management of myofascial trigger points: A systematic review of randomized controlled trials. Complementary Therapies in Medicine. 2017;33:46-57. doi:10.1016/j.ctim.2017.06.003.
32. Jacobs J, Wilson J, Ireland K. Advanced Soft Tissue Release® (ASTR®) Long- and Short-Term Treatment Results for Patients with Neck Pain. MOJ Orthopedics & Rheumatology. 2016;5(4). doi:10.15406/mojor.2016.05.00188.
33. Yuan Q, Wang P, Liu L, et al. Acupuncture for musculoskeletal pain: A meta-analysis and meta-regression of sham-controlled randomized clinical trials. Scientific Reports. 2016;6:30675. doi:10.1038/srep30675.
34. Madsen MV, Gotzsche PC, Hrobjartsson A. Acupuncture treatment for pain: systematic review of randomised clinical trials with acupuncture, placebo acupuncture, and no acupuncture groups. Bmj. 2009;338. doi:10.1136/bmj.a3115.
35. Furlan, Andrea. Systematic review of acupuncture for chronic low-back pain . Japanese Acupuncture and Moxibustion, 2010; .6(1): 37-44
36. Rubinstein SM, Terwee CB, Assendelft WJ, Boer MRD, Tulder MWV. Spinal manipulative therapy for acute low-back pain. Spine. 2011;36(13):825-846. doi:10.1002/14651858.cd008880.pub2.

References

37. Gattie E, Cleland JA, Snodgrass S. The Effectiveness of Trigger Point Dry Needling for Musculoskeletal Conditions by Physical Therapists: A Systematic Review and Meta-analysis. Journal of Orthopaedic & Sports Physical Therapy. 2017;47(3):133-149. doi:10.2519/jospt.2017.7096.

38. Dunning J, Butts R, Mourad F, Young I, Flannagan S, Perreault T. Dry needling: a literature review with implications for clinical practice guidelines. Physical Therapy Reviews. 2014;19(4):252-265. doi:10.1179/1743288x13y.0000000118.

39. Morihisa R Eskew J McNamara A, et al. Dry Needling in subject with muscular trigger points in the lower quarter: a systematic review. Int J Sports Phys Ther. 2016;11(1):1-14.

40. Cotchett MP, Landorf KB, Munteanu SE. Effectiveness of dry needling and injections of myofascial trigger points associated with plantar heel pain: a systematic review. J Foot Ankle Res. 2010;3:18.

41. Cummings TM, White AR. Needling therapies in the management of myofascial trigger point pain: a systematic review.Arch Phys Med Rehabil 2001;82:986-92.

42. Xue CC, Helme RD, Gibson S, et al. Effect of electroacupuncture on opioid consumption in patients with chronic musculoskeletal pain: protocol of a randomised controlled trial. Trials. 2012;13:169. doi:10.1186/1745-6215-13-169.

43. Scott N. A., Guo B., Barton P. M., Gerwin R. D. Trigger point injections for chronic non-malignant musculoskeletal pain: a systematic review. Pain Medicine. 2009;10(1):54–69. doi: 10.1111/j.1526-4637.2008.00526.x.

44. Ernst E, Canter PH. A systematic review of systematic reviews of spinal manipulation. Journal of the Royal Society of Medicine. 2006;99(4):192-196.

45. Young JL, Walker D, Snyder S, Daly K. Thoracic manipulation versus mobilization in patients with mechanical neck pain: a systematic review. J Man Manip Ther. 2014;22:141–153. doi: 10.1179/2042618613Y.0000000043.

46. Filho JCANDS, Gurgel JL, Porto F. Effects of stretching exercises for posture correction: systematic review. Manual Therapy, Posturology & Rehabilitation Journal. 2014;12:200. doi:10.17784/mtprehabjournal.2014.12.200.

47. Thacker SB, Gilchrist J, Stroup DF, Kimsey CD. The Impact of Stretching on Sports Injury Risk: A Systematic Review of the Literature. Medicine & Science in Sports & Exercise. 2004;36(3):371-378. doi:10.1249/01.mss.0000117134.83018.f7.

48. Small K, Naughton LM, Matthews M. A Systematic Review into the Efficacy of Static Stretching as Part of a Warm-Up for the Prevention of Exercise-Related Injury. Research in Sports Medicine. 2008;16(3):213-231. doi:10.1080/15438620802310784.

49. Borchers et al. A Systematic Review of the Effectiveness of Kinesis Taping for Musculoskeletal Injury

50. Gordon R, Bloxham S. A Systematic Review of the Effects of Exercise and Physical Activity on Non-Specific Chronic Low Back Pain. Healthcare. 2016;4(2):22. doi:10.3390/healthcare4020022.

51. Ajimsha M, Al-Mudahka NR, Al-Madzhar J. Effectiveness of myofascial release: Systematic review of randomized controlled trials. Journal of Bodywork and Movement Therapies. 2015;19(1):102-112. doi:10.1016/j.jbmt.2014.06.001.

52. Desmeules et al. Impingement Syndrome: also called Swimmer's Shoulder

References

53. Desmeules FCA, Côté CH, Frémont P. Therapeutic Exercise and Orthopedic Manual Therapy for Impingement Syndrome: A Systematic Review. Clinical Journal of Sport Medicine. 2003;13(3):176-182. doi:10.1097/00042752-200305000-00009.

54. Gross A, Kay TM, Paquin J-P, et al. Exercises for mechanical neck disorders. Cochrane Database of Systematic Reviews. 2015. doi:10.1002/14651858.cd004250.pub5.

55. Saragiotto BT, Maher CG, Yamato TP, et al. Motor control exercise for chronic non-specific low-back pain. Cochrane Database of Systematic Reviews. August 2016. doi:10.1002/14651858.cd012004.

56. Cheatham SW, Kolber MJ, Cain M, et al. The Effects of Self-Myofascial Release Using a Foam Roll or Roller Massager on Joint Range of motion, muscle recovery, and performance: A Systematic Review. International Journal of Sport Physical Therapy. 2015 Nov;10(6):827-38.

57. Castro-Sánchez AMCAD, Matarán-Peñarrocha GA, Arroyo-Morales M, Saavedra-Hernández M, Fernández-Sola C, Moreno-Lorenzo C. Effects of myofascial release techniques on pain, physical function, and postural stability in patients with fibromyalgia: a randomized controlled trial. Clinical Rehabilitation. 2011;25(9):800-813. doi:10.1177/0269215511399476.

58. Furlan A, Yazdi F. Complementary and Alternative Therapies for Back Pain II.

59. Penas C, Campo M. Manual therapies in myofascial trigger point treatment: a systematic review. Journal of Bodywork and Movement Therapies. January 2005.

60. Vernon H, Schneider M. Chiropractic Management of Myofascial Trigger Points and Myofascial Pain Syndrome: A Systematic Review of the Literature. Journal of Manipulative and Physiological Therapeutics Vol 32 Iss 1. January 2009.

61. Kim JH, Lee HS, Park SW. Effects of the active release technique on pain and range of motion of patients with chronic neck pain. Journal of Physical Therapy Science. 2015;27(8):2461-2464. doi:10.1589/jpts.27.2461.

62. Wong CK, Abraham T, Karimi P, Ow-Wing C. Strain counterstrain technique to decrease tender point palpation pain compared to control conditions: a systematic review with meta analysis. Journal of Bodywork and Movement Therapies. 2014 Apr;18(2):16573. doi: 10.1016/j.jbmt.2013.09.010.

63. Jakel A, Von Hauenschild P. A systematic review to evaluate the clinical benefits of craniosacral therapy. Complementary Therapies in Medicine. 2012 Dec;20(6):45665. doi: 10.1016/j.ctim.2012.07.009.

64. Green C, Martin CW, Bassett K, Kazanjian A. A systematic review of craniosacral therapy: biological plausibility, assessment reliability and clinical effectiveness. Complementary Therapies in Medicine. 1999. 7, 201-207

65. Clare A Helen, Adams Roger, Maher G Christoper. A systematic review of efficacy of McKenzie therapy for spinal pain. Australian Journal of Physiotherapy. 2004 Vol. 50.

66. Machado, Luciana Andrade Carneiro; de Souza, Marcelo von Sperling ; Ferreira, Paulo Henrique ; Ferreira, Manuela Loureiro. The McKenzie Method for Low Back Pain: A Systematic Review of the Literature with a Meta-Analysis Approach. April 20th, 2006. Volume 31 - Issue 9 - p E254-E262 doi: 10.1097/01.brs.0000214884.18502.93

67. Ravenek, M. J., Hughes, I. D., Ivanovich, N., Tyrer, K., Desrochers, C., Klinger, L., & Shaw, L. (2010). A systematic review of multidisciplinary outcomes in the management of chronic low back pain. IOS Press. Retrieved from http://web.a.ebscohost.com.vanguard.idm.oclc.org/ehost/

References

pdfviewer/pdfviewer?vid=12&sid=06eb7fdd-c09c-407c-8fae-c12356183f73%40sessionmgr4010.

68. Kaija A Karjalainen MD. Multidisciplinary Biopsychosocial Rehabilitation for Subacute Low Back Pain in Working-Age Adults: A Systematic Review Within the Framework of the Cochrane Collaboration Back Review Group http://journals.lww.com/spinejournal/Abstract/2001/02010/Multidisciplinary_Biopsychosocial_Rehabilitation.11.aspx

69. Maria Ospina, Christa Harstall. Multidisciplinary Pain Programs for Chronic Pain: Evidence from Systematic Reviews. https://www.researchgate.net/publication/237306550_Multidisciplinary_Pain_Programs_for_Chronic_Pain_Evidence_from_Systematic_Reviews

70. Van Geen et al. The Long-term Effect of Multidisciplinary Back Training: A Systematic Review. http://journals.lww.com/spinejournal/Abstract/2007/01150/The_Long_term_Effect_of_Multidisciplinary_Back.17.aspx

71. Wynn, T. A. (2012). Mechanisms of fibrosis: therapeutic translation for fibrotic disease. Nature medicine, 18(7), 1028-1040.

72. Occupational Safety and Health Administration. (n.d.). Computer Workstations eTool: Proper Position. Retrieved from http://www.osha.gov/SLTC/etools/computerworkstations/positions.html[1]

73. Dahlhamer, J. (n.d.). Prevalence of chronic pain and high-impact chronic pain among adults in the U.S. Retrieved from https://consensus.app/papers/prevalence-chronic-pain-highimpact-chronic-pain-among-dahlhamer/

74. Johannes, C. B. (2018). Prevalence of Pain in United States Adults: Results from the Johannes Study. Retrieved from https://consensus.app/papers/prevalence-pain-united-states-adults-results-johannes/

75. Vos, T., Lim, S. S., Abbafati, C., Abbas, K. M., Abbasi, M., Abbasifard, M., ... & Murray, C. J. L. (2018). Global, regional, and national incidence, prevalence, and years lived with disability for 354 diseases and injuries for 195 countries and territories, 1990–2017: a systematic analysis for the Global Burden of Disease Study 2017. The Lancet, 392(10159), 1789-1858. https://doi.org/10.1016/S0140-6736(18)32279-7

76. Hay, S. I., Abajobir, A. A., Abate, K. H., Abbafati, C., Abbas, K. M., Abd-Allah, F., ... & Murray, C. J. L. (2018). Global, regional, and national disability-adjusted life-years (DALYs) for 333 diseases and injuries and healthy life expectancy (HALE) for 195 countries and territories, 1990–2016: a systematic analysis for the Global Burden of Disease Study 2016. The Lancet, 390(10100), 1260-1344. https://doi.org/10.1016/S0140-6736(17)32130-X

77. Rock, K. L., Kono, H. (2008). The inflammatory response to cell death. Annual Review of Pathology: Mechanisms of Disease, 3, 99-126. https://doi.org/10.1146/annurev.pathmechdis.3.121806.151456

78. Hurley ET, Calvo-Munoz I, Desai N, Buckley PS, Tanji JL, Greenbaum BS, Feeley BT. Systematic Review and Meta-Analysis of Nonoperative Platelet-Rich Plasma Shoulder Injections for Rotator Cuff Pathology. Arthroscopy. 2021 Jan;37(1):265-278. doi: 10.1016/j.arthro.2020.08.035. Epub 2020 Sep 11. PMID: 33131197

References

79. Ebadi S, Henschke N, Forogh B, Ansari NN, van Tulder M, Bagheri R, Fallah E. Therapeutic Ultrasound for Chronic Pain Management in Joints: A Systematic Review. Pain Pract. 2020 Apr;20(4):425-442. doi: 10.1111/papr.12864. Epub 2019 Dec 16. PMID: 31095336.

80. Xu C, Michail M, Cheng L, Cheng L, Xie X, Zhang M. A systematic review of clinical studies on electrical stimulation therapy for patients with neurogenic bowel dysfunction after spinal cord injury. Spinal Cord. 2018 Nov;56(11):1059-1073. doi: 10.1038/s41393-018-0180-z. Epub 2018 Aug 10. PMID: 30313096

81. Arroll B, Goodyear-Smith F. Corticosteroid injections for osteoarthritis of the knee: meta-analysis. BMJ. 2004 Apr 10;328(7444):869. doi: 10.1136/bmj.38039.573970.7C. PMID: 15039276; PMCID: PMC387493.

82. Ekhtiari S, Horner NS, Hincapie CA, Aleem AW, Cheng J, Boettner F, Piuzzi NS. Intra-articular saline injection is as effective as corticosteroids, platelet-rich plasma and hyaluronic acid for hip osteoarthritis pain: a systematic review and network meta-analysis of randomised controlled trials. Br J Sports Med. 2021 Mar;55(5):256-263. doi: 10.1136/bjsports-2020-102195. Epub 2020 Aug 10. PMID: 32788249.

83. Conaghan PG, Kloppenburg M. Debate: Intra-articular steroid injections for osteoarthritis – harmful or helpful? Osteoarthritis and Cartilage Open. 2023 Mar;5:100218. doi: 10.1016/j.ocarto.2023.100218

84. Sousa Filho LF, Barbosa Santos MM, dos Santos GHF, Araújo AC, Jennings F, Calders P, Ferreira GE. Corticosteroid injection or dry needling for musculoskeletal pain and disability? A systematic review and GRADE evidence synthesis. Chiropr Man Therap. 2021 Dec 16;29(1):49. doi: 10.1186/s12998-021-00408-y. PMID: 34920524; PMCID: PMC8683524.

85. Coombes BK, Bisset L, Connelly LB, Brooks P, Vicenzino B. Optimising corticosteroid injection for lateral epicondylalgia with the addition of physiotherapy: A protocol for a randomised control trial with placebo comparison. BMC Musculoskelet Disord. 2009 May 7;10:76. doi: 10.1186/1471-2474-10-76. PMID: 19422718; PMCID: PMC2688524.

86. Stecco, C. (2015). Functional Atlas of the Human Fascial System. Churchill Livingstone Elsevier.

87. Stecco, L. (2016). Atlas of Physiology of the Muscular Fascia. Piccin.

88. Bordoni, B., & Zanier, E. (2015). Understanding fibroblasts in order to comprehend the osteopathic treatment of the fascia. *Evidence-Based Complementary and Alternative Medicine, 2015.* https://doi.org/10.1155/2015/860934

89. Gauglitz, G., Korting, H., Pavicic, T., Ruzicka, T., & Jeschke, M. (2011). Hypertrophic scarring and keloids: Pathomechanisms and current and emerging treatment strategies. *Molecular Medicine, 17*(1-2), 113-125. https://doi.org/10.2119/molmed.2009.00153

90. McCulloch, J., & Kloth, L. (2010). Wound Healing: Evidence-Based Management (4th ed.).

91. Bordoni, B., & Zanier, E. (2015). Anatomic connections of the diaphragm: Influence of respiration on the body system. *Journal of Multidisciplinary Healthcare, 8*, 281-291. https://doi.org/10.2147/JMDH.S70111

92. Gauglitz, G. G., Korting, H. C., Pavicic, T., Ruzicka, T., & Jeschke, M. G. (2011). Hypertrophic scarring and keloids: Pathomechanisms and current and emerging treatment strategies. *Molecular Medicine, 17*(1-2), 113-125. https://doi.org/10.2119/molmed.2009.00153

93. Kumka, M., & Bonar, J. (2012). Fascia: A morphological description and classification system based on a literature review. *Journal of the Canadian Chiropractic Association, 56*(3).

References

94. Benjamin, M. (2009). The fascia of the limbs and back. *Journal of Anatomy, 214.* https://doi.org/10.1111/j.1469-7580.2008.01011.x

95. Barnes, J. (1990). *Myofascial Release.* Paoli, PA: John F. Barnes, P.T. and Rehabilitation Services, Inc.

96. Yang, C., Du, Y., Wu, J., et al. (2015). Fascia and Primo Vascular System. *Evidence-Based Complementary and Alternative Medicine, 2015,* 1-6. https://doi.org/10.1155/2015/303769

97. Findley, T. W. (2011). Fascia Research from a Clinician/Scientist's Perspective. *International Journal of Therapeutic Massage and Bodywork, 4*(4), 1-6.

98. Willard, F. H., Vleeming, A., Schuenke, M. D., Danneels, L., & Schleip, R. (2012). The thoracolumbar fascia: Anatomy, function and clinical considerations. *Journal of Anatomy, 221,* 507-536. https://doi.org/10.1111/j.1469-7580.2012.01511.x

99. Fallon, S. (2012). Nourishing Traditions: The Cookbook that Challenges Politically Correct Nutrition and the Diet Dictocrats.

100. Thompson, J. (4th ed.). Nutrition: An Applied Approach.

101. Wilson, J., & Lowery, R. (2017). The Ketogenic Bible: The Authoritative Guide to Ketosis.

102. Mercola, J. (2017). Fat for Fuel: A Revolutionary Diet to Combat Cancer, Boost Brain Power, and Increase Your Energy.

103. Litchford, M. (2012). Nutrition Focused Physical Assessment: Making Clinical Connections.

104. Vasquez, A. (Date not provided). Textbook of Clinical Nutrition and Functional Medicine, Vol. 1: Essential Knowledge for Safe Action and Effective Treatment (Inflammation Mastery & Functional Inflammology).

105. Bennett, P., & Bland, J. (2010). *Textbook of Functional Medicine.*

106. Sanchez A, Reeser JL, Lau HS, Yahiku PY, Willard RE, McMillan PJ, Cho SY, Magie AR, Register UD. Role of sugars in human neutrophilic phagocytosis. Am J Clin Nutr. 1973 Nov;26(11):1180-4. doi: 10.1093/ajcn/26.11.1180. PMID: 4541857.

107. IASTM Image: https://www.temu.com/5pcs-set-stainless-steel-iastm-therapy-massage-tools-tissue-fascia-recovery-muscle-massager-guasha-scraping-gua-sha-massage-tool-g-601099540868938.html?

108. Case Studies Video Link: https://advancedsofttissuerelease.com/treatment-videos-2/

Recommended Resources

How to Access Online Content

1. Open the camera app on your smartphone.
2. Point the camera at the barcode.
3. A notification will appear with a link. Tap the notification to open the link in your browser.

1. Posture and Body Mechanics Training Videos

2. Case Studies and Recorded Live Treatment Videos

3. <u>Limited Time Offer</u>: FREE 30-minute Health Coach Consultation

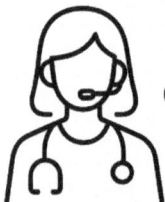